THE POETRY OF NURSING

Literature and Medicine
MARTIN KOHN AND CAROL DONLEY, EDITORS

1. *Literature and Aging: An Anthology*
   EDITED BY MARTIN KOHN, CAROL DONLEY, AND DELESE WEAR

2. *The Tyranny of the Normal: An Anthology*
   EDITED BY CAROL DONLEY AND SHERYL BUCKLEY

3. *What's Normal? Narratives of Mental and Emotional Disorders*
   EDITED BY CAROL DONLEY AND SHERYL BUCKLEY

4. *Recognitions: Doctors and Their Stories*
   EDITED BY CAROL DONLEY AND MARTIN KOHN

5. *Chekhov's Doctors: A Collection of Chekhov's Medical Tales*
   EDITED BY JACK COULEHAN

6. *Tenderly Lift Me: Nurses Honored, Celebrated, and Remembered*
   BY JEANNE BRYNER

7. *The Poetry of Nursing: Poems and Commentaries of Leading Nurse-Poets*
   EDITED BY JUDY SCHAEFER

8. *Our Human Hearts: A Medical and Cultural Journey*
   BY ALBERT HOWARD CARTER III

The
Poetry of Nursing

Poems and Commentaries of

Leading Nurse-Poets

Edited by Judy Schaefer

The Kent State

University Press

KENT, OHIO

© 2006 by The Kent State University Press, Kent, Ohio 44242
Library of Congress Catalog Card Number 2005018966
ISBN 978-0-87338-848-1
Manufactured in the United States of America

10 09 08 07 06   5 4 3 2 1

Library of Congress Cataloging-in-Publication Data

The poetry of nursing : poems and commentaries of leading nurse-poets /
edited by Judy Schaefer.
p. cm. — (Literature and medicine series)
ISBN-13: 978-0-87338-848-1 (pbk. : alk. paper) ∞
ISBN-10: 0-87338-848-8 (pbk. : alk. paper) ∞
1. Nurses' writings, American.   2. Nurses' writings, American—History
and criticism.   3. Poets, American—20th century—Biography.
4. Nurses—United States—Biography.   5. American poetry—20th century.
6. Nurse and patient—Poetry.   7. Nursing—Poetry.   8. Nurses—Poetry.
I. Schaefer, Judy, 1944–   II. Literature and medicine (Kent, Ohio) ; 7.
PS591.N8P64 2005   811'.508092161073—dc22   2005018966
British Library Cataloging-in-Publication data are available.

For my husband, Dan.

And with gratitude to Joanne Trautmann Banks
and to Drs. Jane and Lawrence Kienle,
The Doctors Kienle Center for Humanistic Medicine,
The Pennsylvania State University College of Medicine, Hershey.

Contents

❦

Introduction

༄

JUDY SCHAEFER

THE STRONG VERTEBRAL COLUMNS of nurses form the infrastructure of the modern health-care system. These are the women and men who are my heroes: nurses whose magic is healing wounds and sorting out the trail of tubes and catheters; nurses who empty the drains that empty from your colon, your bladder, your chest—from your anywhere—where sludge has built up and caused you pain; nurses who help you heal, keep you safe with pen lights through the pain of night, and in the morning pull you fresh from the bedcovers. Nurses will keep your secrets safe; they will host your spouse, your lover, and your friend, treat them all the same, and never reveal names. Nurses preside at the feast of tea and toast, Jell-O, and milk and graham crackers—and NPO (Nil Per Os or nothing by mouth). They hold your hand and stroke your brow when visiting hours are done. They help you die in peace, holding you until you are gone and keeping you in the pockets of their hearts forever. Twenty-four hours a day, seven days a week, and three hundred and sixty-five days a year, through holidays, snow, and rain—nurses! 24/7/365!

The storehouse of stories and experiences is rich for a nurse. The nurse-poets in this book represent a spectrum of nurses who are writing professionally as well as creatively in prose and poetry, and this is but the tip of a poetic iceberg that crackles with new and ancient energy. Cortney Davis and I had the privilege of editing two international anthologies of creative writing by registered nurses, *Between the Heartbeats* (1995) and *Intensive Care* (2003). This book is an extension of those books; the brave nurse-poets represented here witness and give linguistic reference to pain and thereby start a new discourse. When asked who I read routinely, I answer, "My fellow poets." Theirs are the poems I love.

Rare is the opportunity to read both the poem and the poet's commentary. I know—or think I know—the process and some of the reasoning behind my own poems. Yet, I realize I know little about the process of my fellow nurse-poets. In the past decade, nurse-poets have risen to a level of comfort in "having a say," in breaking and decoding the stenotic silence. My impression is that a certain amount of courage is involved.

Elaine Scarry, in *The Body in Pain,* (New York: Oxford University Press, 1985, p. 4) writes, "Whatever pain achieves, it achieves in part through its unsharability, and it ensures this unsharability through its resistance to language." Pain, felt and observed, she says, "does not simply resist language but actively destroys it." Although the band of nurse-writers is increasing, and many nurses have written without indicating their nursehood, I often wonder why more nurses, who know the troubled health-care system so well, are not writing. Scarry suggests it is the pain, witnessed and inflicted in the name of treatment and cure, that resists language.

To give linguistic reference starts a process—a discourse. The written word and the writing of words can have a healing influence for both the writer and the reader. While I personally want to create literary art, I also know that the process is healing for me. I think it has, in the past and now, made me a better nurse. Some bold examples of linguistic reference are in the following poems: *cigarette burns on a child* in Deppe's "Admission, Children's Unit," *helplessness* in Ebner's "Daily Activity Log," *dehiscence* in Haddad's "Dehiscence," *death by cancer* in Masson's "Metastasis," *anger* in Mercer's "Exiles," *death of our own loved ones* in Nealon's "Human-Headed Bull below Empty Space," *the almost dead* in Sergi's "Home Visits," *separation* in Sievers' "Holding On," *a father's drinking* in Webster's "The House on Bolton Road."

My own "Who Owns the Libretto?" is an analysis of narrative ownership from the parents' viewpoint. It provides a learning opportunity for me and, also, the poem raises the question of who owns the story.

WHO OWNS THE LIBRETTO?

They browsed quickly through
The medical stacks
Text after text
Pushing page after page
He watched her quick movements
He held her gray coat
To allow her armroom
And give her space to breathe
She pulled from
Shelf after shelf

Bent on her knees
Stretched up her arms
Then leaned back and sat down
Lifted her knees as in
Stirrup for childbirth
Book after hardbound book
Looking for a gush of water
Found one
This one
Splash of a waterfall
Look at this one
Pointed him to it
The illness there
Their respirations now fast
The illness of their child
Described with paragraphical details
Graphs and diagrams
Percentages and prognoses
They looked
Side to side
Held their breath
So as not to be caught
In their act
Not to be scolded

This poem is imaginative and "made up" but was inspired by a team of clinicians, me included, wondering about a particular patient's need and right—imagine, right—to go to the stacks and read the medical texts. Right? Curiously, this poem was written prior to the explosion of available knowledge on the Internet. The parents in this poem would now be at home with their personal computer. The poem, published originally in 1993 in *Wild Onions* (literary journal of Penn State University's College of Medicine) and then, in 1995, anthologized in *Between the Heartbeats*, is already dated and obsolete.

In "Who Owns the Libretto?" I "try on" the perspective of the parents. Patients we see in their white-sheeted beds and on the exam-table paper are much more complex and have much richer lives than we can comprehend in fifteen-minute time slots. While giving linguistic reference to the parents' need to know, I am also giving the "words" back to the patient and the parents, returning the words, "The Libretto," to the source, so to speak.

ZONA PELLUCIDA

The bar is packed
chairs overfilled
Strum of laughter and conversation
Clink of glasses, guitar
Hallway and wall space
teaming with eager contestants
Her cups runneth over;
That one in her hand
and those two in her bodice.
Her skirts touching, swaying
legs rubbing, inviting
Hardly noticeable, cellular rituals
                Hardly noticeable

except to designated-driver wives
who have cars already parked
in their zona pellucida

The cellular basis, hormonal and enzymatic, of who and what we are is fascinating. Emotion combined with science is compelling. In my imagination I can freely examine intimacy. "Zona Pellucida" reflects my own feeling of being the onlooker. Either as young Judy Welker at the high school prom in 1962 in Missouri or adult Judy Schaefer in a pub in Ireland, I am the historian. I expect many nurses are the designated drivers of their world. You know what I mean, a look that occurs between nurses in a moment of crisis that says, "We can handle this." We can, and do. The nurse-poet goes a step further and tells the rest of the world about it through literary devices such as metaphor and simile.

MATHEMATICS

I don't give advice anymore
in conversations seeking advice.
I keep my watch on home time.
I deduct or add as I go
relative to where I am.
While you chat of pain, betrayals,
I look at my watch—face of Pythagoras.
You intuit impatience

You stop—abrupt. I want to apologize.
I'm reminded that it is the end of the day, somewhere:
>   A soldier dies in unoccupied territory on a peace mission
>   A three-year-old ceases-to-breathe for random reasons
>   on a gurney in LA
>   A vintner in Sonoma goes to the cellar to test the cabernet
>   My father lights his pipe and prepares to dream in Missouri
>   My mother fluffs his dream like a comforter filled
>   with new goose down
>   My son-in-law talks to his son through my daughter's belly
>   My husband lights a cigar on Blue Mountain and pours cognac
>   A watchman on Cutter three-seventy-nine watches the sea
>   with electronic eyes
>   A bartender in Killybegs has locked the door, gone home
>   An old priest in Rheims, unable to sleep, prepares
>   a funeral mass
I am reminded, as you talk, that we have all the time we need.
I wonder how to live; I wonder how to die.
But that is not the question you ask.
I want to talk about watches; the mathematics of this point in time,
trains that arrive and the purchase of the rare crystal ball.
I won't give advice anymore.

There is that pure desire to produce a poem that will ring so true that—ping—the glass is shattered. If I had that wish come true, it would be for this poem. Though it is a poem of the imagination, the protagonist is me. While in a job that required traveling, I was always trying to stay on hometown-time, wondering what everyone was doing at that moment. While everyone at the airline counter recognized me, my yellow cat did not. Flowers would bloom in the garden and I would miss them. Grandchildren were growing. I eventually gave up this job and came home. Ironically, it was beginning to sink in: life was short. If life is lived fully, however, one has all the time needed. Ironic; life is short, but we have all the time we need.

Yet, having said all such sensible words as I have in "Mathematics," a nurse wants—really wants—to give advice. Nurses develop a modicum of wisdom over time and most find it difficult to restrain themselves. It is so easy for the nurse to insert an opinion. I want to diagnose, label, plan for care, and implement that plan. I can, and do. "I won't give advice anymore," while a statement, is also a mantra to keep my mouth shut and my hands to myself.

An empowered and functionally oriented mythology is evolving to replace our much-loved but dated and passive symbols such as the nurse's cap and the white uniform. Myth works metaphorically and functionally on a subconscious level of a deeply embedded and long-held belief in a particular story or parable. Ironically, the new mythology evidenced here is closer to the art of nursing as described in 1860 by Florence Nightingale in her hands-on book, *Notes on Nursing*. Consider, for instance, the real and metaphoric function of *pockets* in Davis's "The Nurse's Pockets," *patient* in Rosenzweig's "Crossing the Field," *plastic bag* in Spencer's "Army Nurses, Vietnam, 1966," and *hands* in Studer's "Higher Learning" and in Bryner's "In Praise of Hands." Descriptive symbols of evolving functional nursing mythology!

The fourteen major nurse-poets here, born in different geographical locations and with different clinical backgrounds, have been poets since childhood. They all carry journals or bits of paper in their pockets, always ready to have a say about what they witness in their work or in their private lives. I have written a brief introduction for each nurse-poet's section. Names have been changed and appropriate consent obtained for these poems and commentaries to protect individual privacy. We pass the baton, shift to shift and generation to generation. I pass the baton to the poets here and to all the others represented by this band of bards. You know who you are.

POETRY PUBLICATIONS

Schaefer's poetry publications include the following books:

Between the Heartbeats: Poetry and Prose by Nurses. Co-editor. Iowa City: Univ. of Iowa Press, 1995. The first anthology of creative writing by registered nurses.
Harvesting the Dew. Long Branch, N.J.: Vista, 1997. A poetry collection.
Intensive Care: More Poetry and Prose by Nurses. Co-editor. Iowa City: Univ. of Iowa Press, 2003.
The Porch Went all around the Blindman's House. Chapbook. 1983. Self-published as a gift for daughter.

Schaefer has poems published in the following journals:

Academic Medicine; American Journal of Nursing; Apprise; Harrisburg Review; Clinician Reviews; Health Affairs; Journal of Medical Humanities; The Lancet; Literature and Medicine; Mediphors; Wild Onions.

Schaefer's poetry is included in the following anthologies:

Between the Heartbeats: Poetry and Prose by Nurses. Ed. Cortney Davis and Judy Schaefer. Iowa City: Univ. of Iowa Press, 1995.

Intensive Care: More Poetry and Prose by Nurses. Ed. Cortney Davis and Judy
    Schaefer. Iowa City: Univ. of Iowa Press, 2003.

A Life in Medicine. Ed. Robert Coles and Randy Testa. New York: New Press,
    2002.

Ten Years of Medicine and the Arts. Ed. Lisa Dittrich. Washington, D.C.:
    Association of American Medical Colleges, 2001.

Word of Mouth. Ed. Kaye Roberts. Langollen, Wales: Poetry Today, 1998.

Jeanne Bryner

ℰ

Bryner's poems are bold and muscular. The imagery in Bryner's powerful poems pushes, pulls, and carries. The movement is both cerebral and vertebral, as demonstrated in "Siderails" when she tells us that second-year nursing students can perform the mental work of "figure[ing] doses [and] write[ing] care plans," as well as the physical work of "wipe[ing] the silver rails clean again." In another poem she writes about coal miners and "the weight / of picks slung over our shoulders." In these lines, particularly in the word "weight," the reader recognizes both the reality of the miners' work and the implications of this trade: the working conditions, the health risks, the economic hardship. By the time we come to the end of Bryner's essay, we are not surprised to learn that she is an emergency room nurse—all action and speed. If we are hurt and on an emergency room litter, this is the language we want. She will speak for us—if we cannot.

WHEN I STUDY MY COLLECTION of poems, those published and those not yet published, one theme threads the quilt: whose hands hold the reins of power. Whether I'm examining my Appalachian family's migration, the perception of medicine's hierarchy, the respect for the workings of the human body, or the angst of balancing the many roles of being a woman, words are the ladders my people climb to wave their arms wildly from the rooftops. This metaphorical ladder may be a poem, letter, essay, or piece of fiction. I try to speak for lives surrounded by the flood of silence: *Here, over here. Look at us for a moment. Listen to what we have to say.*

Writing lets me speak in a bold voice I cannot wrestle forth in any other way. It allows me to sass and show the world that I don't need big words to say that we all need grit to survive this journey. Though it is difficult to convince people, all of our lives are extraordinary and deserve some form of documentation. No one has had an easy life. For years, my friend tried to make the raisin oatmeal cookies she remembered from her childhood. She bought cookie cookbooks, women's magazines filled with cookie recipes, and the fair cookbook. All of the cookies were good and grainy, but none were the ones she tasted as a girl. One Tuesday, she pulled the oatmeal box from her own cupboard, lifted its lid, found the recipe printed on it, and went to work. Her bright kitchen filled with the warm smell of sweetness, and when she sampled the cookies, they were right. They were the ones she loved as a girl. We can search here and there and everywhere for the best, but the best is not *out there*. What we are really looking for, I believe, is a way to honor and celebrate the work of our life.

Grief and love, struggle and hope are the many sides to one boulder. Every day, we push the boulder up Hope's mountain, and while we sleep, it rolls back down, finds its way to the muddy creek. Every nursing shift fills with emotions, but where is the ledger to document how nurses turn chaos into order? In nursing we learn, *if it isn't documented, it never happened*. With that in mind, I don't want to ignore my lived experiences of bedside nursing care, being a daughter, wife, mother, teacher, sister, and writer. These are the spokes to the wheel of my life. To ignore one weakens the balance of my existence. I hold on to poetry the way a drowning person clings to a floating tree branch. I choose to speak honestly and clearly about all I have seen and heard and felt as a woman who carries the stories of her people inside her heart and a nurse who bears the yoke of a stethoscope around her neck.

I was born to a family of storytellers and fiddlers, farmers and coal miners, to women who knew how to birth their babies at home and not scream out in pain. I would take my seat beside them and sit quietly, listening to those who preached. I do not know why I am the one carrying stories in my head and writing them down as poetry. I just know if I don't write things down, I feel like my breasts are full and there's no baby to nurse. I have to write the way I have to breathe. I know how lungs can stiffen from silt, how men die from what they cannot cough up. My father was a coal miner; he suffered from black lung. My brother is a coal miner. My family's drilling rigs sunk the shaft in Pennsylvania where nine miners were rescued from the Quecreek Mine in 2002. While at Bucknell University in 1992, I wrote the following poem to honor working-class lives.

COAL MINER, CAPLES, WV, 1938

Consider this coal miner, who is still young
and blue-eyed, how he rests his jaw
in timbers of his palm, face dusted over
with what most shafts exhale.

Down the road you know there's a shot hole,
the place where he drags his hope like a sledge
past the sun's pajamas, and pulleys lower
him in a wire basket.

Inside dark caverns, lessons begin.
His common hands follow glistening layers
of pigment to the middle ear of the mountain.
What does he hear in this immense labyrinth?

Does his heart complain that his shovel holds
no ruby, that air dances, a full-breasted woman
who spins her ether, drips juices over him,
a siren's song to make him stay?

He carries a silver pail, jam bread, yellow
cheese, coffee, cold in a jar, the memory
of screech owls in the hollows of his boyhood,
where he runs, fearless, and magnolias hang

in pink ruffles, warm yams stick to his fork.
He tastes all of this, smells brown manure
falling from his father's mules. His vision
persists, a grail filled with morning stars.

Think of the way we are all porters, the weight
of picks slung over our shoulders, leaving
in darkness, morning after morning, the shimming
up of our thigh bones to hold us in stanchions.

Isn't this it? The fatigue, days of garrets
furnished in quiet grumbles. Yet, we are rich
as this miner who scoops black honey
from a nettled ridge. We become the bear, reign
supreme in the starless land of tunnels,
where men with lanterns are kings.

By the time I wrote this poem, I had practiced nursing for over a decade.
Notice the images of ether and sleep. A nurse understands how medicine
can suspend time and pain. One evening while waiting in our library for my

daughter to check out her books, I picked up a *Life* magazine, started turning pages. Marion Post Wolcott's photos of coal camps, miners, and Appalachian women looked up at me. I knew these faces. The blackened face of the miner spoke to me. The small girl carrying the kerosene in the half-light just before dawn reminded me of my cousins, sisters, and me. I dug change from my purse and copied the pages. I wrote a series of poems from these photos. One of them was "Coal Miner, Caples, WV, 1938." My youngest brother lives less than a half mile from Caples, West Virginia.

Eleven years after my first published poem, I finally started exploring and celebrating my Appalachian heritage. Thanks to encouragement from college professors and writing teachers, I shared pieces of writing about my nursing life. The writing was declared *poetry,* and one of my professors named me a *poet.* This language gave me wings. In a voice so unlike my early rhyming poems, I begin to say who I was and where I came from without reservation. I examined my people, my work, and patients' lives. I learned to know myself better and discovered the value of mining memory.

Still, there is a strong message in my culture: *don't get above your raisin'.* It is well known yet unspoken, like many societal rules. Nursing has historically been a woman's profession, and the numbers continue to remain lopsided with regard to gender. Culture influences how we respond to authority figures, and in Appalachia, I believe, only a preacher would be more revered than a physician. The preacher is entrusted with our souls, the physician, with our bodies. When all home remedies failed, it was time to travel to town, visit the trusted family physician. However, when my mama was birthing her children in my granny's bedroom, it was a nurse who boiled water, held things together during labor, and snipped the cord. She lived across the creek, two farms past my granny's. It was she who spanked the babies, massaged mama's uterus, and handed the local physician a pen to sign birth certificates. Birthing is a natural process, and this labor was sacred, done by women who knew they could never take credit for it.

So many elements of illness are mysterious. Why do we really get sick? And why do some of us get well while others perish? Why can't we say how we really feel about dying to our families? Why can't families share how they feel about watching us suffer? What is the power of this experience that makes language fail us? How can we build a bridge across the silences? These questions haunt and challenge nurses to find ways to facilitate language, facilitate healing. First as a student nurse and now a practicing nurse, every day I learn more about grief and the delegation of truth. Here is an early poem about truth in the country of illness. It is a poem about the powers of observation, the delicacy of interpersonal relationships, and acceptance of duty.

SIDERAILS

Dr. Stanislaw, did you know
second-year nursing students
are only permitted to speak
when asked a question,
attempt venipunctures
if veins resemble sewer pipes,
and make rounds holding hands
with head nurses?

Second-year blue uniforms
have the bath down pat,
can figure doses, write care plans
that instructors scar

with red slash marks.
One Friday morning, I made rounds
with you and Miss Kitch on 6 East.
A family member asked you to please
inform your silver-headed patient,
Miss Farley, that they could not possibly
care for her any longer, and a nursing home
was the only answer.

We pulled the curtain; you lifted
her blue-print gown, exposing
a sagging yeast-dough belly
now held fast with black suture
railroad crossings, a penrose drain—
everything healing well,
and then your hands gripped
her cool siderails, knuckles white:
Your family doesn't feel
capable, the best place, where you'll get
good care, a nursing home after you're
discharged from here.

This was the dirty work
I didn't know

surgeons had to do.
I think damp rails
will snap because your knuckles
are blanched so—your voice slices
syllables—steady, scalpel thin.

You wish this molasses quiet
was a rotten-meat gallbladder,
a ruptured spleen, anything
you could cut away.

Miss Farley weeps,
soft, Baptist tears.
For an eyelash moment,
you hold her hand.

On hairpin ceiling track,
shushed curtain slides,
Miss Kitch sniffs, carries the chart,
and I want to tell you—something,
standing under pure white and black
clock hands weaving our gray lives
into honest shawls, I'd like to say,

Man, that was a shit deal
and you got class Doc,
but I'm a second-year nursing student.
You are Chief of Surgery.
No one asked me for an answer.
I'm just here to learn
how 70% alcohol and ten Hail Marys
wipe silver rails clean again.

As I grow older, I appreciate more and more the house of my body. It has creaky floors, leaky ceilings, secret hallways and two porthole windows facing the sea. Behind me, the girl I was swings in the backyard and splashes her brothers with water from the garden hose; she runs to catch raindrops in her mouth and rides her bike until dark. There is no way to tell her about what lies ahead: how her mother will die young and her father will suffer a stroke. There is no way to prepare her for the news of infertility, her husband's heart condition, and her daughter's bone tumors. A huge forest stands and waits for the girl. She must walk among the trees, some giving shade and others choked with poison vines. Here she will meet grief and know it as a lifelong companion. She will pass through fire and survive. In the quiet of evening, she will watch others on their journey and learn to love her own life more.

Being around bodies in pain and in various stages of healing, I recognize how hard the body works to repair itself and stay well. I can think of no other machine so amazing in its parts. One night, my husband and I went to see "The Grapes of Wrath" on stage in Cleveland. Steinbeck's characters were as compelling in the theater as I remembered them on the page. Due to arthritis, my husband was barely able to clap. I studied his swollen fingers lying quietly in his lap. I started thinking deeply about his hands and all they had given to make our family unit work. This is one of my favorite poems, and it was written for David's years of hard labor.

IN PRAISE OF HANDS

That they are slaves.
That each tendon's a rope
and the knuckles are pulleys.
That their white bones
line up like pieces of broken chalk.

They are bound by flesh
as leather around a Bible.
That they dance and write
in air the story
of what is lost, what is gained.

That they are soldiers
cut and bleeding, a link
to the heart's kingdom.
That they are so beautiful
a moon has landed on each finger.

That they are trained
for harps and hired for murder.
That the cuticles are shaped
like soft horseshoes.
They contain rivers.

That the ring finger's shyness
suffers when gripped by the powerful.
That the palm yields to blisters
and wears the calloused rags
of repetition.

That they are mythical
with their lifeline's hieroglyphics.
That they struggle
because of their great strength.
They are able to heal themselves.

That they know what it means
to draw the water
and work without pay.
That they will hide our eyes
and pray for our sins.

That they may lift the hammer
and lead our bodies to grace.
That they will make a print
like no other
until they wave goodbye.

In the best of all worlds, art should provoke discussion and new avenues for
thinking. We need to look closely at what is familiar and discover its deep-
est meaning. Mushrooms under a microscope appear to be flower blooms.
Hands held up side by side resemble a menorah. What happens when a
finger/candle suffers a traumatic amputation? All light is needed. A physical
therapist might write a poem for hands, or an orthopedic surgeon, but they
didn't. A nurse chants the body's intimacies because she pilots thousands
of patients in her lifetime. People trust her to facilitate a safe landing. She
catches vomit in towels, cleans blood splashes from her shoes, and pays
attention to the body and its language. An editor asked me, "Why praise the
hands hired for murder?" and I replied, "We need to consider why those
hands were for sale."

People who don't know me well look puzzled when I tell them I'm a
nurse and writer. They often gush with the overused phrase, "I think that's *so
interesting.*" Then, I proceed to tell them much of nursing is observation and
documentation. I think it helps demystify the notion of nurse-authors. Also,

I remind them that physicians have been respected as writers for centuries. Of course, I quickly note that most physicians *have wives*. Nurses now have automatic washers, and during the spin cycle, well now, there are a *great many* opportunities to write and participate in classes for creative writing.

In an effort to grow as an artist, I mine imagination and do research. A book in progress titled *The Good Blue Plates* tells the story of my Appalachian grandparents, who were farmers. A symbiotic relationship exists between the land and farmers: for the purple flowers to open, ants must crawl across the buds, eating the sap. I hope to show the universality of planting and weeding and fretting over a harvest which may or may not succeed.

Metaphorically speaking, we are all farmers pushing different plows, watching patterns of clouds, and hoping for a bountiful crop. It is a never-ending prayer to the Goddess of Harvest: *let my life be fruitful and my years plentiful.* Alone in my study, writing becomes a bridge where I can move back and forth in time and space. I speak with the dead and living and crippled as equals, remember and retell hardships in details gleaned from the couch of real life and the lazy bed of dreams. Reading books for research, I become a child again, sitting in the laps of women and men from other eras and different cultures. Their voices lull and intoxicate me to believe what they say is real.

For six and a half years, I tended to the interviews, poems, and photographs for my book about historical and contemporary nurses, *Tenderly Lift Me.* No writing project in my life demanded more commitment. While initially working on it as a creative writing thesis with a mentor and friend, Maggie Anderson, I pushed many boundaries and discovered new depths to translating lived experiences into poetry. Later, I decided to extend the project to include contemporary nurses' lives. A writing fellowship from the Ohio Arts Council provided me with the opportunity to conduct interviews and research. My sabbatical from hospital nursing was a *lady's agreement* with my director of nursing: I would work one weekend a month for three months. In the best universe, I would have welcomed more time off, more hours to gather interviews, but the nursing shortage dictates the lives of women, directors, and staff nurses. I said to myself, *this book will be my dissertation to the world.*

Created in bits and pieces, I felt the passion of being a partner to my art, living with the process, loving it completely and unconditionally. I began to think in terms of a future where the words I chose to put on paper would stand for my life. It humbled me. I approached language with a fresh reverence and the lives I lifted up for examination with a new and deeper respect. Here, in the negative space, I would sculpt with my bare hands the clay of other people's lives. From the country of the long dead, I would lift nurses, dust them off, and wait for their lips to open. I was transfixed and transported by the poignant moments of these nurses' lives. In draft after draft I honed the poems to be as luminous as the lives they represented. My wastebasket overflowed with failed attempts to paint the murals properly. The nurses' stories became the air filling my nostrils. They became my lost sisters, my brother, returned from a far country. The wars they went through and the scars of their bodies were visceral to me. I could smell the rotting flesh beneath those old bandages and feel the sorry ache of their bones not wanting to move their bodies forward. I wept at my desk and felt no shame. Somehow, this calling became a village in the country of my life. I have never felt so clear about the purpose of writing, recovering, and discovering the truth of other nurses' lives.

There are days when it is truly hectic to straddle the world of nursing and poetry. I work part time and try to maintain high nursing standards. I don't want a weekend warrior nurse caring for me or mine, so I try to provide my patients with a real nurse who happens to write poetry and stories. I never dreamed I could write and publish poems and stories. I never thought I would teach creative writing to others. A firm believer in the healing power of language, I work with cancer support groups, the elderly, school-age children, and any population hungry for what language provides. I insist that student writing be documented in books or booklets, depending on the funds available for publication. Being a teacher has been a huge blessing and privilege. It allows me to show others how to become a good steward to language. My life is full of many miracles and more than a few heartaches. I urge women especially to document their stories and the story of their people. Two-thirds of the world's illiterate population are women. Those are songs, poems, plays, and novels we will never hear. Considering that cacophony of silence, I refuse to feel guilty about one moment spent writing or reading or revising. Let the angel of guilt pass over my house; the blood of my sisters' stilled voices is painted above its blistered white lintel. We all stand on the shoulders of others. To honor the lives of my grandmothers and great-grandmothers whose stories are whispers in the dark, I offer this closing poem from *The Good Blue Plates.*

EARLY FARMING WOMAN

This is not the rainy season.

Across the river, we eye each other,
the dark-skinned man, a bloody lamb
slung over his spear, me with a basket

of seeds, my three children, hungry.
Near our village, water holes shrunk
to puddles, game driven off, bones,
bones everywhere. Four months ago,
my man went with the others

following the scent of rain. He fell
out of a tree, the wind left his body.
I have his arrows, a sliver of flint,
his ear braided in my hair.

We live on land no one else wants,
the men hunt, the women gather.
From stalks, I strip the grain
with my bare hands. They are rough

as bark and seldom suffer.
The man speaks, and it's the sound
of morning birds. My children wave
to him, point to his lamb.

I am tired of dry seeds and praying
for the clouds to tell their story.
I've had my fill of beatings,
carrying the elders' water in clay vessels

Whatever this man wants, I will give him
and my children will eat.
Tonight, they will sleep,
they will sleep and dream.

Poetry is not a china teacup to be lifted and sipped with one's pinky extended.
No. Real poetry opens doors and windows to mansions, madhouses, and mud
huts. Wherever men and women sit in a circle and speak communally, the
songs of our lives are born. Those who are called to speak must lift bandages
to describe the wounds' terrible beauty. For lives surrounded by the flood of
silence, mine as well as others, poetry becomes a footbridge strong enough
to carry us all.

Poetry Publications

Bryner's poetry publications include the following books:

Blind Horse. Huron, Ohio: Bottom Dog, 1999.
Breathless. Kent, Ohio: Kent State Univ. Press, 1995.
Not Far from Town. Chapbook. 2003. Self-published as a gift for husband.
Saguaro. Chapbook. 2000. Self-published as a gift for daughter.
Tenderly Lift Me. Kent, Ohio: Kent State Univ. Press, 2004.

Bryner has poems published in the following journals:

Allegheny Review; American Journal of Nursing; Analecta; Annals of Internal Medicine; Appalachian Heritage; Black Warrior Review; Cream City Review; Creative Nursing; Dickinson Review; 5 AM; Geriatric Nursing; Hawaii Review; International Journal of Arts Medicine; The Journal; Journal of Emergency Medicine; Journal of Emergency Nursing; Journal of Holistic Nursing; Journal of Kentucky Studies; Journal of Medical Humanities; Kaleidoscope: International Magazine of Literature, Fine Arts, and Disabilities; Kestrel Lullwater Review; Minnesota Review; Negative Capability; Now and Then; Prairie Schooner; Poetry East: Poem; Red Brick Review; Sou'wester; Texas Journal of Women and the Law; Viet Nam Generation; West Branch; Wind; Wittenberg Review.

Bryner's poetry is included in the following anthologies:

Are You Experienced? Baby Boom Poets at Midlife. Ed. Pamela Gemin. Iowa
   City: Univ. of Iowa Press, 2003.
Between the Heartbeats: Poetry and Prose by Nurses. Ed. Cortney Davis and
   Judy Schaefer. Iowa City: Univ. of Iowa Press, 1995.
Boomer Girls: Poems by Women from the Baby Boomer Generation. Ed. Pamela
   Gemin and Paula Sergi. Iowa City: Univ. of Iowa Press, 1999.
Cancer Poetry Project: Poems by Cancer Patients and Those Who Love Them.
   Ed. Karin B. Miller. Minneapolis: Fairview, 2001.
A Gathering of Poets. Ed. Maggie Anderson and Alex Gildzen. Kent, Ohio:
   Kent State Univ. Press, 1991.
The HeART of Nursing: Expressions of Creative Art in Nursing. Ed. M. Cecilia
   Wendler. Indianapolis: Center for Nursing, 2002.
Intensive Care: More Poetry and Prose by Nurses. Ed. Cortney Davis and Judy
   Schaefer. Iowa City: Univ. of Iowa Press, 2003.

Learning by Heart: Contemporary American Poetry about School. Ed. Maggie Anderson and David Hassler. Iowa City: Univ. of Iowa Press, 1999.

A Life in Medicine: A Literary Anthology. Ed. Robert Coles and Randy Testa. New York: New Press, 2002.

Literature, Class, and Culture. Ed. Paul Lauter and Ann Fitzgerald. New York: Addison, Wesley, Longman: 2001.

On Being a Doctor 2: Voices of Physicians and Patients. Ed. Michael A. LaCombe. Philadelphia: ACP, 2000.

Sweeping Beauty: Contemporary Women Poets on Housework. Ed. Pamela Gemin. Iowa City: Univ. of Iowa Press, 2005.

What's Become of Eden: Poems of Family at Century's End. Ed. Stephanie Strickland. Tarrytown, N.Y.: Slapering Hol Press, 1994.

Cortney Davis

෫ଚ

In "The Nurse's Pockets" Davis writes about an asset that is crucial to the nursing profession. No nurse believes that he or she can function, really function, without the "pocket" of the uniform and the "pocket" of the heart. With candid poetry like Davis's the nursing profession will develop symbols to replace those that are beginning to slip into a loving and historic past, such as the nursing cap and white uniform. Fresh, functional symbols, such as "pocket" with its double implications, support a new nursing mythology of hands-on action. In "Heroics" the new myth is at work. The nurse is a decisive and intimate figure, no longer the white angel hovering and distant. In the new mythology, the nurse is in the action. These are bold, new poems that expand the language of nursing and lead the profession into a new millennium.

WHEN I WAS LITTLE MORE than a year old, my mother's dormant tuberculosis flared and my father, just home from Italy at the end of World War II, was suffering from terrible nightmares—what we'd now call post-traumatic stress syndrome. My parents decided I would be better off in a healthier environment and sent me to live with their best friends, the Coles, a couple with two children of their own, a boy and a girl.

I became the Coles' second daughter and the baby of the family. As months went by (the Coles would write to me many years later), I seemed to forget my parents. Nevertheless, they said, I was never quite at home in my new family. In a photo from that time, I'm sitting on my surrogate mother's lap, straining toward the camera as if I might catch sight of someone I know in the lens. Mrs. Cole holds me tight and her two children smile at me, but I'm flailing my arms, trying to escape, my brow fixed in a frown.

After I turned two, after I learned to talk, after living with the Coles for almost as long as I'd lived with my parents, my mother and father came to reclaim me. My mother's health had improved, although she'd still depend on a nanny to help with my care, and my father had found a job and seemed to be coping with his nightmares. Once again, I switched families. My parents told me I readjusted quickly. However, for a long time I couldn't tolerate the slightest separation. If my mother turned the corner in a grocery store, out of sight only for a moment, I would fall to the floor screaming, thinking she was gone forever.

Once I was reunited with my family, my childhood was for the most part happy and constant, yet I never quite got over the sense that someone I loved might, at any minute, disappear. Encouraged by my father and compelled by what he called my "imagination of disaster"—a trait we shared—I began to write poems, a perfect way to reexperience and make sense of the world and my place within it. Soon, when I wasn't reading, I was writing. I learned that writing holds on to things, and it also lets them go. It allows you to change the outcome of events. It gives you wings and, at the same time, binds you to reality. Writing encourages you to pay attention with all your senses. The images in your mind come to life when you see, touch, taste, smell, and hear them, then transfer those sensations in precise language to the blank page. I learned that when you write, you stumble upon metaphors that allow you to describe even the most abstract emotions in concrete words.

From an early age, I assumed that I'd grow up to be a writer—that's the path I followed until I married, had two children, and then divorced. There wasn't much money to be earned by writing and, a single mother, I urgently needed a *real* occupation. When a friend encouraged me to become a nurse's aide (with on-the-job paid training and flexible shifts), I jumped at the opportunity. As years went by and my children grew, I moved up the career ladder from nurse's aide to OR tech to RN, along the way abandoning my writing and forgetting the magic and the urgency of poetry.

After graduating from an associate-degree nursing program, I worked first in intensive care, then as a head nurse in oncology. At the same time, I enrolled in the local university to complete my BS in nursing. But when I took a class in contemporary poetry, my long-suppressed impulse to capture experiences in the written word resurfaced. My teacher, a poet in his fifties, was living proof that one could be a parent, hold down a job, and also be a writer. Suddenly, as if given permission, I began to write poems again. Everything became "material"—my childhood, my children, the strangers I saw in town, the owls that hooted in our trees at night. But I never wrote about nursing. What I did in my professional life seemed out of bounds, too clinical, too separate from my "other" life.

Then I met Toby, a young woman dying of leukemia.

Toby was a patient on our oncology floor off and on for more than four years. She and I looked alike: brown hair, blues eyes, and freckles. We each had two children the same ages, a girl and a boy. The doctors on the oncology ward kept mixing up our names, calling me Toby and her Cory, my nickname. Neither of us minded—in fact, for fun, we joined in. Hi Cory, I'd say to her. Hi Toby, she'd answer back, confusing the doctors even more. Then, during what we thought was a routine admission, on a Sunday when her husband and children were out of town for the day, Toby died. There were three of us at her bedside: me, her doctor, and a respiratory therapist.

For months, I couldn't get the image of Toby, dying, out of my mind. I didn't know what to do with my grief, a loss I couldn't, it seemed, share with anyone. After all, patients died every day. And, as another nurse reminded me, Toby hadn't been, not really, a personal friend. But the loss I felt was palpable.

Faced once again with the task of making sense of the pain of separation, I wrote a poem about Toby. Writing it allowed me to discharge my feelings of personal sorrow and professional inadequacy in the face of her illness. The poem became a way to let Toby go and, paradoxically, a way to hold on to her memory forever. Writing that poem rekindled the mystery of writing for me; I was reminded that when you think you can't find the right words to say something, that's where poetry begins.

I've been writing about my work and my patients ever since. When I write, poetry and nursing merge—a poem becomes the place in which the act of caring becomes a way of keeping, and the mysteries of our world are revealed in the sensual reality of physical detail. For me, nursing is intimate, tactile, spiritual, and utterly unlike any other way we humans have of caring for one another. Nursing is not mothering and yet shares some of mothering's traits. Nursing is not doctoring, even though nurses are as essential to a patient's well-being and recovery as a physician. Nursing is not friendship or love, yet many nurses do love their patients, just as patients often love their nurses. And in nursing—just as in mothering, friendship, or love—we must, sooner or later, confront the reality of separation, even when that separation is accompanied by joy. We nurses tend our patients, and they always leave us. Some go home, cured, and we celebrate their leaving; others die, and we remember them. I tried to capture the unique way nurses care for their patients—sure to lose them and yet privileged to become the guardians of their memories—in my poem, "The Nurse's Pockets."

The narrative of this poem is familiar to most nurses: A patient is dying. His doctor, having arrived to deliver this message, has a hard time breaking the news. He stalls outside the door. The patient has to confront him: "So doc, what's the verdict?"

The patient's response is typical, individual, human—he thinks about his good life; he worries about the cat that will be left behind. When the doctor leaves, the nurse enters. Devoid of any miracle cures, perhaps not even privy to every aspect of the patient's medical course, she already knows the patient is dying. All she can offer are her bare hands and her presence. She stays with the patient, doesn't ask anything of him, and offers what she can: "the sound of water / wrung from the warm washcloth, / the smell of yellow soap." She *tends* the patient physically, and her tending brings comfort.

For me, the heart of caregiving—its astonishing intimacy and privilege—is summed up in the poem's next two lines: "—she spends time praising / the valley of his clavicle, his hollow mouth." The nurse's ministrations are akin to praise: she acknowledges even the smallest human detail, in a sense blessing the patient for the journey to come. She marvels at the secrets of the body, the "valley of the clavicle." She praises the patient's "hollow mouth," conjuring not only the image of a dying patient's gaping lips but also of the absence of words. How many times, caring for a patient, does a nurse stand in silence, letting his or her hands convey what speech cannot? How many times does a patient, contemplating death in the company of his nurse, find that words are unnecessary? The nurse spends time with the patient, thankful for the opportunity to serve in such an uncluttered and honest way, sharing the moment when two human beings stand before the certainty of death and yet still honor the gift of life.

When the nurse returns the next morning, her patient has died. His bed is empty except for the map of his body still pressed into the sheets, the "depression" he leaves behind: not only the physical indentation in the hospital bed, but also the terrible absence in the minds and hearts of those who knew or loved him. The nurse, cleaning up, gathers the only evidence she has of his existence: old gumdrops in his drawer, "A comb / woven with light hair, and a book / with certain pages marked." She hides these in her pockets and takes them home, placing them in a trunk for safekeeping. In fact, "She has trunks in every room of her home, / full of such ordinary things." Perhaps all those trunks are like poems. Whenever she wants, she can open one up and recall, from those ordinary things, the unique life of each individual patient.

We nurses are masters of the art of separation. We remember our patients. We remember most readily those whose recoveries we've witnessed and those who we've accompanied toward death—a journey entrusted specifically to nurses. Poetry captures, for me, every nuance of caregiving: the wonder of birth; the reality of death; the sorrows sometimes too deep to talk about; the revelations that occur, often like lightning, sometimes more quietly, during the most unexpected moments, as when a nurse is bathing a patient, silently, and all of her history and all of his meet in the space of that interaction.

The Nurse's Pockets

When patients are told they're dying
they say something simple:
I've had a good life or *Who will feed my cats?*
It seems harder on the doctor—
he waits outside the door, stalling,
until the patient confronts him.
So, Doc, they say. *What's the verdict?*

Soon, a nurse comes to bathe the patient.
There is only the sound of water
wrung from the warm washcloth,
the smell of yellow soap,
and the way she spends time praising
the valley of his clavicle, his hollow mouth.

Then, a morning when the patient leaves,
taking his body. The nurse finds nothing
but the bed with its depression,
its map of sheets she strips.
In the drawer, gumdrops. A comb
woven with light hair, and a book
with certain pages marked.

She takes all these into her pockets.
She has trunks in every room of her home,
full of such ordinary things.

My first job after graduating from nursing school in 1972 was in the coronary care unit in a small Connecticut hospital. Our unit had seven beds fanned out around the nurses' station like spokes on a wheel. Only two of us stood guard on the night shift, me and a nurse's aide who covered her head with a bath blanket and slept until 4 A.M., when she'd suddenly wake, hurrying to bathe patients and set them up for morning rounds. Because there was no house staff, residents from New York's Columbia Hospital would moonlight in the CCU. Like me, the residents were young and eager to experience everything—the dramatic codes, the odd illnesses, the heroic rescues. Sometimes the resident and I would watch the monitors at the nurse's desk, half wishing for and half dreading the moment when *something* would happen.

My poem "Heroics" is about that time in a young caregiver's career—that foolish time when we see a patient's disease more clearly than we see the patient, when even the disease seems disconnected from the patient, becoming something we borrow to hold up, examine, and read about. If we're lucky, we'll discover a disease that's unusual and fascinating, something to talk about in the cafeteria and on rounds.

The poem's first two stanzas set the scene—a nurse in the CCU, watching the monitors. In response to a "fractious pattern of impending doom," she goes to the patient's bedside, laying her hands on the man's arm to comfort him. At the same time, she scans the monitor screen, almost hoping to see the "rare but cherished run of ventricular fib." The curtain is closed; the patient's body is "silvered" by light filtering though the IV bottle. The nurse is conflicted. The man in the bed is real and suffering. But, like "the snake at Eden's gate," the possibility of *action, drama, the opportunity for heroics* tempts her.

When the patient's heart dies, the nurse and the resident come to life. They love the adrenaline rush, the militarylike precision of actions well rehearsed and performed with the best intent. The team places the paddles like "two cold palms" on the patient's chest; they "hit" again and again until the "heart's muscle heaves and wobbles on." The patient is saved. Time for reflection will come later.

The next morning, the nurse completes the mundane task of taping monitor strips into the patient's chart, reexperiencing the moments when the "patient died, then, where we arrived." In the background, she hears the "saved man sing." Looking up at the monitor, she sees "his heart's line burn." Only then does she grasp the magnitude of what has occurred. She has witnessed a "solar eclipse"—an act not only beyond her control but also beyond her understanding and, for the patient, a primal, life-altering event. The poem's last line hints at a newly felt humility, one tinged with fear. The saving of this patient was something she "dared" to watch with her "bare eyes," a moment that has burned into her consciousness and left her unprotected, vulnerable, and, probably, a better nurse.

Is there a time when, as beginners, we *should* love that heroic moment? Can we admit or accept such an odd and seemingly undesirable trait in medical and nursing students, in ourselves? Can we talk about it? Certainly as we gain experience, we *see* differently. Our patients become more and more like us. Their diseases become ours. As our life stories blend with those of our patients, heroics is not so much a matter of rushing to the bedside and performing a miracle as it is having the endurance to stay the course: to minister to patients in small, daily ways; to understand that our journey is to the *patient,* and the disease is only a gate we must go through to reach our destination.

When nurses and doctors read this poem, there might be two reactions. Some will ask, "How can a nurse possibly say such things?" Others might admit that they too have felt the thrill of discovering a "fascinoma" or the addictive energy of running to a code. Ideally, young practitioners could explore both points of view. Selfless giving *and* self-conscious detachment are both part of a learning process that culminates in a mature approach to caregiving—that looking again with "bare" eyes, the humility with which we dare to care for our fellow human beings.

HEROICS

I love a slight tremor on the screen,
a waver in the complex that signifies a restless patient
or the fractious pattern of impending doom.

Behind drawn curtains, I touch the patient's body
silvered by the IV bottle's light. *Are you*
all right? I ask, and watch the bedside monitor's
silent sweep, searching for PVCs, SVT,
or the rare but cherished run of ventricular fib,
the snake at Eden's gate.

Most of all, I love when the heart's undulating line
goes flat, triggering a high-pitched whine
that doesn't stop until we pop all electrodes
from the patient's chest, slather the metallic paddles
like two cold palms and snug them tight against his bone.

Hit! we shout, and *Hit again!*
until the heart's muscle heaves and wobbles on.

The next morning, I Scotch tape monitor strips
across the chart to demonstrate where the patient died,
then, where we arrived. I listen
to the saved man sing, and see his heart's line burn—
a solar eclipse I dared to watch with my bare eyes.

In holocaust survivor and contemporary novelist Elie Wiesel's book *The Night Trilogy: Night, Dawn, The Accident* (New York: Hill and Wang, 1985, p. 237), a man has been hit by a car and now lies in his hospital bed. A nurse comes to give him injections against the pain. He can't open his eyes to see her, but he imagines she must be beautiful. As the nurse strokes his face, he wonders if she will kiss him, a "little meaningless kiss on the forehead." He thinks to himself, "*A good nurse kisses her patients when she says good night.*"

The image of a nurse bending over her patient and kissing him stayed in my mind. I wondered about the nature of caregiving, the *intent* of caregivers. A poem, "The Good Nurse," evolved in response to the image evoked by Wiesel's novel. I tried to stay with this image and let the details unfold as they might.

As the poem begins, the nurse is thankful for her patients' daily, recurring needs: the positioning of bodies, the straightening of sheets. The intimacy of these ministrations seems the province of nurses or mothers, and indeed they are part of my personal nursing experience. In the third stanza, the nurse quells the patient's thirst by offering her own cold glass and, in order to relieve the patient's discomfort, she extends her own fingertip to the "bee," metaphorically taking the pain into herself. This desire to diminish a patient's suffering, even to shoulder suffering in place of that patient, is the province of all caregivers.

As the poem unfolds, the image of "mothering" becomes stronger and more literal, and the constancy and minutiae of caregiving becomes counterpoint to changes in the nurse's "real" world. Her children have grown up, moved away. Unable to "bind them" in her arms, unable to force constancy into her own world or into the world of her children, she turns to patients. Patients, she knows, will always need their caregivers. The poem discovers that caregivers will always need their patients.

The nurse's caring, however, is not motivated by love for her patient, at least not the kind of love we share with family and friends. This nurse has chosen a profession that expresses caring through recurring, intimate actions. Like every caregiver, she balances the inconsistencies of life against the certainty of loss and death. She "kisses" her patient as he goes into a realm known to her, so far, only by its modifiers: the patient's cyanotic skin, the death stare. Like any "good" caregiver, physician or nurse, she knows she too will enter this realm some day, and her kiss sends the patient on his way with a special, fearful, human benediction.

As I reconsidered this poem with writing this commentary in mind, more questions arose. How would a physician begin a poem about caregiving, and for what would he or she be grateful? Is a chaste kiss—or the manner of caring it suggests—something a patient might also expect from a "good" doctor? And as we, nurses and physicians both, grow and change in our personal lives, as we release patients to health or to illness, what is it about caregiving that represents, at least to me, the greatest constancy of which humans are capable?

The Good Nurse

A good nurse kisses her patient
when she says good night.
—ELIE WIESEL

Our kiss is in gratitude
for rumpled sheets, the hourly
turning of patients. For pillows
placed between legs,

cotton booties pulled over raw heels
and in thanksgiving
for the patients' needs:
Their thirst quelled

by our cold glass.
Their pain,
sharp and relentless as a bee
charmed by our fingertips.

The kiss has everything to do
with sons who look at us
and disappear, daughters
who line their eyes with blue

and borrow our too-loud laughter.
We want to bind them
in our arms. Instead, we tend
the patient who longs for us.

He knows we will rush to him,
stroking his earlobe, kissing lightly
his eyelid, his cheek—
not for love,

but for what is constant:
The way skin hurries
to bruise, and the last gaze
freezes the mind.

Poems usually come, for me at least, when two different ideas collide, knocking against each other and causing sparks. I might be driving in my car, listening to NPR, or in the grocery store, or in the middle of doing a patient's exam, when suddenly someone will say something, or there will be a certain feel to the breeze, or I'll notice a certain expression flit across my patient's face and *bam,* I know there's a poem in the making.

At first, I may only be aware that two different but somehow related images or thoughts have come to mind. For example, I might see the way my patient's finger traces the words on page and, out of nowhere, recall the way my mother, when she was losing her eyesight, would run her fingers over everything, trying to identify fabric, shape, and size. Or I might be at the beach, vacationing, when I see a mother lift her toddler, saving him from the hot sand, and immediately think of my father, dying, and how the hospice nurse told me she was giving him morphine to "carry him over his pain." Perhaps because I'm both nurse and poet, my everyday experiences provide rich material, and this unexpected coming together of two ideas happens often.

I can tell the ideas are genuine, headed for a poem, if they hang around, whispering about in my brain and refusing to be forgotten. I find myself ruminating about the events those ideas evoke, recalling nuances of sound, sight, taste, and smell, or the way something felt beneath my hand. Then, after a period of gestation, the impulse to *write* becomes so urgent that I know the poem's birth is imminent.

I've said "period of gestation" and "birth" and, in a way, this coming together of two disparate ideas is like the merger of egg and sperm. Two totally unlike entities join and over a period of time create a third being with a life of its own—for our purposes, a poem that may bear little resemblance to the two impulses that set its creation in motion. Like the nine months of gestation, sometimes the path from that first clanging together of two different ideas to the actual completion of the poem can be prolonged and difficult. Other times, the waiting time is shorter, the delivery easier. Rarely, a poem appears fully formed, ready to get up and start running on its own.

The creation and delivery of "Everything in Life Is Divided" fell somewhere in between: the poem didn't have a long gestation, but it would hardly qualify as one of those miracle births either. The initial idea for the poem (that clashing together of different thoughts) came to me as I stood in the hallway after attending a poetry reading. A friend paused to say hello. We chatted about how much we'd enjoyed the reading. He asked after my own writing, then said something like, "It must be hard for you to divide your life between nursing and poetry." *Bam.* I got that here-comes-a-poem feeling, as if I might open my hands and find one idea—how my life is divided between the clinical and the creative—in one palm, and another idea—how my love and attention was divided at the time of my first grandchild's birth—in the other. I didn't know where that second idea came from. Was the memory of my daughter's labor and delivery stirred by something the poet had read? Was it something my friend said, something insignificant and now forgotten? Was it simply that the memory of my daughter giving birth was always with me, and when I thought about my divided life, the computer in my brain called up other instances of division? I don't know if a poet can name the exact origin of the creative impulse, any more than a painter or composer or novelist can. But it's always cause for celebration when such ideas arise.

I kept talking to my friend in the corridor, but inside, my mind was humming. When he walked away, I took paper and pen from my pocketbook and jotted down the words "Everything in Life is Divided." Then I wrote "poetry and nursing / labor room." When I got home, I put the slip of paper near my computer.

For the next several days, I thought about those two ideas. I didn't think about them *rigorously*, like I might think about learning the newest treatment for hypertension or the latest recommendations for prenatal testing. Instead, I thought about them creatively, letting them hang around with me while I went to work, folded laundry, ate dinner. The two ideas lived with me, and their heartbeats—that internal sense of rhythm and line—grew stronger and stronger. Finally, when I had a whole morning to write, I sat down at the computer. On the blank, white screen, I typed what I already knew would be the title: "Everything in Life Is Divided." Then I waited.

I find that something quite magical happens when I sit down, ready to write. My thoughts wander, yet in some way my mind becomes razor sharp, ready to catch images, to call memories up from the cellar of my subconscious, and to suspend logical thinking, or at least to suspend the kind of thinking that judges and hinders. My fingers, poised over the computer keys, become a conduit. Some energy, some force, gathers in the deepest recesses of my brain and travels, like electricity, down my arms, through my wrists, and into my fingertips. I type out lines and images and all the things that *come to me*. It's not like being in a daze or being drugged or drunk—it's as if I'm totally and completely awake, in synch, and ready to catch the poem as it hurls itself, squalling, onto the page.

As I wrote this poem, images and words and ideas about all the things that might be divided came to mind. I thought about night and day, about the ocean and the shore; then I remembered vacationing with my husband at Martha's Vineyard, how the sand became the barrier between us on our blanket and the sea. Perhaps because I was thinking about the blanket (and that reminded me of a picnic), the image of the apple appeared—Adam and Eve?—and I could picture the apple sliced in two, the way the black seeds stand out against the fruit's white flesh like a two-sided Rorschach. Of course, since my vocation is nursing, I thought about the body, the way our organs are partitioned, the way our physical selves guide our lives toward suffering or rejoicing, tragedy or comedy—the double-headed "possibilities of the Greek mask."

Pausing at my computer, I looked around and saw, on one side of my desk, a pile of half-written poems; on the other side, some nursing texts, waiting to be read. Ah, I thought, the core idea, the thing that started the poem going in the first place. I had come to the point that occurs in every poem, the place where something has to happen, something has to take off. *Now,* my brain seemed to signal, *now* it's time to bring in that moment in the delivery room when, after my first granddaughter was born, my own daughter was hemorrhaging. Standing by her side, I lost any semblance of medical knowledge or experience and became simply a mother, frightened to death that my daughter wouldn't stop bleeding, and so unable to turn my attention to the healthy, crying newborn across the room. Birth is another division; I realized how all of life revolves around the two polarities, Joy and Fear, that faced me that night in the delivery room. I had to balance them, as we all have to balance them every day. Then, my daughter's bleeding stopped.

Well, in retrospect, writing the poem sounds a bit easier than it was.

Like any newborn, my poem had to be cleaned up, wiped off, examined. The initial delivery of words to the page might resemble nothing more than a blob of images, a random collection of memories, a few unfinished sentences. Like the nurse in the nursery, the poet has work to do. Once the baby is born, the nurse has to administer certain medications, monitor vital signs, observe how the infant acclimates. The poet has to turn an eye to revision—the looking again at the initial impulse and the resulting collection of words, perhaps the most essential part of writing. Word choice, simile, metaphor, tense, line breaks, grammar, logic, rhythm, and rhyme are only a few of the technical considerations that help turn that word-blob into a poem that might transcend the initial, personal impulse and reach a more universal audience.

In first draft, "Everything in Life Is Divided" was twice as long. I'd written on and on, bringing into the poem my deceased mother, having her look into the incubator and join hands with me and my daughter. I described the Greek masks, comedy and tragedy, and I used four-line stanzas rather than the spare couplets of the version here. I struggled with grammar in the tricky second and third stanzas, making sure that the reader could tell who was being separated from whom and by what. I cut about five or six stanzas, words and images that didn't really belong in this poem at all. Finally, I tinkered, reading the poem out loud, changing line breaks and altering word order, eliminating unnecessary words and polishing punctuation.

Is the poem finished? One of my poetry teachers, Honor Moore, said that poems are never finished, merely "excused." In some ways, having a poem published excuses it—it leaves home and goes out into the world to be read and judged by others. In other ways, poems never leave their poets. We tuck them in our sleeves, if only in memory, and we recall how they came to be, a process that required, like all wonderful pursuits, our full attention and devotion, the capacity to be surprised, the willingness to work hard and, ultimately, the ability to juggle the various aspects of our lives and our selves and find the right words to bring them together.

Everything in Life Is Divided

Everything in life is divided:
twenty-four hours that fade from day to night,

the sand at Martha's Vineyard, where we vacationed last year,
separating us from the ocean

where we swam, then returned to our blanket,
the two of us making one marriage,

sharing the apple sliced to reveal the identical
black seeds of its surprised face.

Even our bodies can be halved, although less evenly:
lungs partitioned into lobes, the heart's blood

pumped from right to left, the brain's two hemispheres
directing our arms, our legs,

our lives into the two possibilities of the Greek mask.
My life's work, too, is divided—

on one side of my desk, unfinished poems;
on the other, nursing books with dog-eared pages.

Aren't we all somehow divided?
Like when my daughter was in labor, my first

grandchild emerging into the room's blue air,
suddenly entering new territory,

and how, when after the delivery my daughter kept bleeding,
I couldn't look at the newborn in the incubator

but stood fast beside my child, the woman who once
slipped from my life into her own and now had divided herself again

while I balanced in my hands *Joy* and *Fear,* cradling them both
until the bleeding stopped.

Like other nurses, I'm no stranger to death. If you work in our field long enough, no matter where you're employed or where your ambition takes you, sooner or later you'll be called upon to sit with the sick, the grieving, the dying. Perhaps those of us who do our nursing in places like the intensive care unit or the cancer ward sit with the dying and the grieving more often. But eventually, this task comes to us all.

The first time I saw a dead person I was a nurse's aide, my first evening on the job. The charge nurse had asked me to make vital-signs rounds, which meant going from room to room and taking the patients' temperatures, pulses, and blood pressures. I set off with my clipboard and a stethoscope, feeling a bit awkward in my new blue pinafore apron and white shoes, a scissors tucked into my pocket. At first, everything went fine. I introduced myself and chatted with patients, some in double rooms, some in eight-bed wards. I'd take a patient's glass thermometer from the bedside plastic holder, wipe off the alcohol (I can still smell the sharp, silver smell of it), shake down the glittery column of mercury, and place the glass rod under the patient's tongue. While the thermometer "cooked," I held the patient's wrist and counted the heartbeats for one minute. Like most of the other aides, I fudged on the respirations, writing down "20" for each patient. It wasn't until later, when I became an RN like the nurses I admired—the women in white, the ones who soothed patients with a word or a gesture, the ones who knew how to insert intravenous lines and how to shock patients back to life—that I learned that ten or twelve breaths an hour was the norm. That night, it was Mr. Tonelli's obvious lack of breathing that caught my eye.

When I pulled back his curtain and called, "Good evening! Here to take your blood pressure," he didn't answer. Flat on his back, gaze fixed on the overhead light, the old man had died with his mouth open, a dark "O" underneath the overhang of his boney nose. Something seemed missing, as if whatever made him Mr. Tonelli had gotten up and left, abandoning the unbreathing husk of his body for me to find. His skin was gray, shriveled, and dry to my one-finger touch. In an instant, I recognized *dead*. Dead as my gerbil had been when I was six, dead as all those goldfish floating sideways at the top of the tanks of my childhood, dead as the puppy I'd seen hit by a car when I was ten. One minute, a body could be full and soft and illuminated by something that was, without a doubt, life; the next minute, that same body could be sunken, inexplicably smaller, and dim, as if there were indeed a radiant soul that had been called away.

I stood for a moment, staring at Mr. Tonelli. I stroked the veiny back of his hand. I felt his hard yellow nails. I touched his bare arm with the back of my hand, as if checking a baby's bath water. I leaned over to peer into his eyes, blue and sunken into their orbits. I remember saying a prayer, something like "Please let his soul rest in heaven in peace." I took a deep breath, as if for both of us, and sat down next to him on the bed. I'd never met Mr. Tonelli before, yet I was the first one to see him like this. It seemed an honor beyond words.

When I left his room to walk back and deliver the news to the charge nurse, I was changed. I'd seen death, *human* death. And while this man's body had something in common with the other dead bodies I'd seen, it was astoundingly different. I told the nurse, and she seemed to cave in a bit, as if someone in her keeping had slipped away unaccompanied, and this brought her pain. Looking back, I know how many deaths she must have seen, how many bodies she'd bathed and wrapped and walked to the morgue, how many families she'd called or sat with or cried with. She straightened her shoulders. "Was this your first?" she asked.

It wasn't until many years later that I experienced the *process* of dying, a patient's actual passage from this world to the next. Being present during the dying is not like coming in after, when the storm has passed and everything is quiet. Dying, especially what hospice nurses call "the active phase," is not easy to witness. A patient may be awake, talking and twisting, sweating, apparently fighting. They might be semi-aware, gasping for air, suddenly opening their eyes and staring at you just at the moment their hearts freeze midbeat, their lungs stop billowing in and out. Or they could be totally comatose, dying privately, without giving us witnesses any hint of farewell. After Mr. Tonelli, after I'd become a registered nurse, after I'd sat with a few dying patients, my experience with death seemed never ending, as if death recognized that I'd somehow earned my stripes in *being there*. Death took every opportunity to call me back into the room, and death threw everything at me: the kind of final hemorrhage we call "bleeding out"; burned, broken or drowned children; postpartum mothers, their milk just coming in, who died of ruptured aneurysms; old women who smiled as they departed, mocking death and helping me to smile too. Let death do what it will, I told myself. It's my job, it's my calling, *to stay.*

Stay I did, but always afraid, always with my heart pounding so mightily that it could have pumped the blood for both of us, me and my dying patient. Sometimes I felt as if I would faint or become ill; sometimes I felt the presence of God; sometimes I felt the room electric with spirits; and sometimes I felt that the dying person was paying attention, living every moment, dragging death out because being *here* was so precious. Other times I felt patients hurrying to leave, sadly turning their backs. A few times, death felt dangerous and overpowering. Every time, I studied what was happening like a novitiate. I didn't know then for what I was practicing.

My mother died in 1991, in a nursing home bed at 9:30 in the evening. My father slumped, overwhelmed, in a chair nearby. I sat on my mother's bed, as I'd sat on so many patients' beds, holding her hand. The weight of everyone's expectations—my father's; the floor nurses' who knew that because I was there, they could be elsewhere; my own—was a heavy burden. Because I was a nurse, everyone assumed I'd be brave, able to stay and somehow orchestrate this moment for all of us. But, I wanted to shout, This time is different—*This is my mother.* I wanted to run out to my car or sit in the waiting room. I wanted the luxury of saying, "I can't do this." At the same time, I wanted to be there. I *can* do this, I told myself; I've done this so many times before. Inside, I felt terrified and unprepared.

Some years after my mother's death, I wrote this poem. I was able to give voice to that "double vision" I'd experienced at her bedside—part of me her daughter, part of me a nurse—as I stroked her hair, recognized the final heart beat, and said, over and over, that we were there, that we would walk with her all the way. In the poem, I tried to put into words what it's like for any of us nurses to be there at the moment a loved one dies. I wanted to talk about how difficult it is to be both caregiver and family member, both experienced at death and yet, every time, newly come to its bedside.

Something else happened in the process of writing about being present at my mother's death. I let go of much of the terror that being with the dying can awaken in me. I began to see beyond the many individual deaths I've witnessed to the greater arc we call the life cycle, that continuous coming and going. I began to *feel* the rightness of it, the comfort of it; I began to understand that all my patients, my parents, my loved ones, myself, are a part of this continuum. Because I could believe in that glorious, forever-spinning cycle, I stopped believing in death.

I don't know if other nurses feel this way. I don't know if this is something that comes with age and maturity to all of us, or if it's only felt by those who've done their apprenticeships at the bedsides of the dying.

How I'm Able to Love

I'm stunned by death's absence,
by the flesh that remains, changed and yet hardly so.
I try to pretend the body's a pod or insect shell,
but attending the body after death

I see the body with all its attributions
for the first time, totally honest—
a time to satisfy that final curiosity,
the long gaze that reveals a life compressed, unalterable.

Beyond the window, rain falls. Streets below
shine like an untied black ribbon.
When my mother died, I was the one
part nurse, part daughter. I caught her last heartbeat

with my fingertips, knowing that the lungs
fail a few beats after, then breath empties them.
From long experience, I stood at the moment
just before and stroked her hair

as life moved through her as it always does—
pulling itself up through the ankles
through the bruised aorta
taking the heartbeat along, gathering the last

lungful of air and leaving nothing, all this
up through the jaw and, at the moment life breaks free,
out the open eyes. The hands respond,
as if the body wasn't robbed, but had been clinging and let go.

I don't believe in death.
Even when the body mottles, even
in its closed casket, I see the body I have touched,
staring at it as I work. Only my fingers

retain the memory
of my memory. This compression is good:
it makes room for all the dead I know and don't know—
the familiar dead and the dead yet to be born.

An inexplicable urge to explore, record, recall, remember, and understand the small, elusive moments of life through language compels me to write. I began writing poems when I was about eight or nine years old; I even have a few scraps of writing (silly poems and awkwardly printed "stories") from when I was six or seven.

As I grew, I read and was in love with Poe, Blake, *Madame Bovary* and *The Scarlet Letter,* W. H. Hudson's magical *Green Mansions,* the poems of Robert Frost and Edna St. Vincent Millay. I loved to listen to my father's retelling and reading-out-loud of Emerson's essays. Our house was filled with books, classic authors next to contemporary writers and serious tomes next to collections of jokes or sociologic studies. I remember one of those, a study of why children played certain games, which I found fascinating—what we did, even in play, had meaning! Everything in life mattered! In early adolescence, I stumbled upon Hemingway, T. S. Eliot, Shakespeare, Dickinson, Whitman, Jack London: I was learning that specific language and sensual imagery were beautiful, and primary to vivid communication.

We also had magazines galore. *The New Yorker* was my favorite. I thought that it was slick and sophisticated, and I loved the wry cartoons, the glamor- ous ads, and the complicated poems and stories. I loved the articles, stories, and photos in *Life* magazine and the Norman Rockwell covers of *Saturday Evening Post.* I read everything I could get my hands on. At breakfast, if I didn't have a book or magazine, I read the cereal boxes. My father, who had been a newspaper reporter, was alert to the many textures of the written and spoken word, to imagery, to language's power to liberate and enchant as well as its ability to deceive, sway, and confuse. My mother loved poetry—I still have one of her favorite volumes, pages marked. My parents and I often discussed language; early on, I learned that words are magic keys, opening our lives to depth, pleasure, and mystery.

POETRY PUBLICATIONS

Davis's poetry publications include the following books:

Between the Heartbeats: Poetry and Prose by Nurses. Co-editor. Iowa City: Univ. of Iowa Press, 1995.

The Body Flute. Chapbook. Easthampton, Mass.: Adastra, 1994.
Details of Flesh. Corvallis, Ore.: Calyx, 1997.
Intensive Care: More Poetry and Prose by Nurses. Co-editor. Iowa City: Univ. of Iowa Press, 1995.
Leopold's Maneuvers. Lincoln: Univ. of Nebraska Press, 2004.
Willy Nilly: Poems for Children. Chapbook. Concord, Calif.: Small Poetry, 2000.

Davis has poems published in the following journals:

Academic Medicine; Alaska Quarterly Review; Amaranth; American Journal of Nursing; Annals of Internal Medicine; Antigonish Review; Bellevue Literary Review; Calyx: A Journal of Art and Literature by Women; Clackamas Literary Review; Conatus; Connecticut River Review; Contexts: A Forum for Medical Humanities; Courrier International; Crazyhorse; Embers; Hanging Loose; Heliotrope; Hobo Jungle; Hudson Review; International Journal of Arts and Medicine; Kaleidoscope: International Magazine of Literature, Fine Arts, and Disability; Kalliope; Journal of the American Medical Association; Journal of Emergency Medicine; Journal of Medical Humanities; Lancet; Litchfield County Times; Literature and Medicine; Massachusetts Review; Ms.; New York Times; Nursing and Health; Care Perspectives; Ontario Review; Pikestaff Forum; Pivot; Poet and Critic; Poetry; Poetry East; Poets On; Prairie Schooner; Reflections on Nursing: The Journal of the Sigma Theta Tau International Honor Society of Nursing; River City; Second Glance; Sentence: A Journal of Prose Poetry; Sifrut; Slow Dancer; Sojourner; The Sun; 13th Moon; Underwood Review; Viet Nam Generation; Witness; Women's Review of Books; Yankee; YearOne.

Davis's poetry is included in the following anthologies:

The Arduous Touch: Women's Voices in Health Care. Ed. Amy Haddad and Kate Brown. West Lafayette, Ind.: Purdue Univ. Press, 1999.
Are You Experienced? Baby Boom Poets at Midlife. Ed. Pamela Gemin. Iowa City: Univ. of Iowa Press, 2003.
Articulations: The Body and Illness in Poetry. Ed. Jon Mukand. Iowa City: Univ. of Iowa Press, 1994.
Between the Heartbeats: Poetry and Prose by Nurses. Ed. Cortney Davis and Judy Schaefer. Iowa City: Univ. of Iowa Press, 1995.
Bittersweet Legacy: Creative Responses to the Holocaust. Ed. Cynthia Brody. New York: Univ. Press of America, 2001.
Cracking the Earth. Ed. Beverly McFarland, et al. Corvallis, Ore.: Calyx, 2001.

Family Reunion: Poems about Parenting Grown Children. Ed. Sondra Zeiden-
   stein. Litchfield, Conn.: Chicory Blue, 2003.
A Fierce Brightness: Twenty-five Years of Women's Poetry. Ed. Margarita Donnelly,
   Beverly McFarland, and Micki Reaman. Corvallis, Ore.: Calyx, 2002.
Grow Old along with Me. Ed. Sandra Martz. Watsonville, Calif.: Papier Mache,
   1996.
In My Life: Encounters with the Beatles. Ed. Robert Cording, Shelli Jankowski-
   Smith, and E. J. Miller Laino. New York: Fromm International, 1998.
Intensive Care: More Poetry and Prose by Nurses. Ed. Cortney Davis and Judy
   Schaefer. Iowa City: Univ. of Iowa Press, 2003.
A Life in Medicine. Ed. Robert Coes and Randy Testa. New York: New Press,
   2002.
Mourning Our Mothers. Ed. Carole Stasiowski. Hartford, Conn.: Andrew
   Mountain, 1998.
Poetry from Sojourner: A Feminist Anthology. Ed. Ruth Lepson. Champaign,
   Ill.: Univ. of Illinois Press, 2004.
Ten Years of Medicine and the Arts. Ed. Lisa Dittrich. Washington, D.C.: Asso-
   ciation of American Medical Colleges, 2001.
Truth and Lies: An Anthology of Poems. Ed. Patrice Vecchione. New York:
   Henry Holt, 2001.
Uncharted Lines: Poetry from the American Medical Association. Ed. Charlene
   Breedlove. Albany, Calif.: Boaz, 1998.

Davis has contributed to the following texts:

Editor's Choices from the Literature, Arts, and Medicine Database. Ed. Felice
   Aull. New York: New York Univ. School of Medicine, 2003.
From Clinic to Classroom: Medical Education and Moral Education. Ed. Howard
   Radest. Westport, Conn.: Praeger, 2000.
Grief and the Healing Arts: Creativity as Therapy. Ed. Sandra Bertman. Ami-
   tyville, N.Y.: Baywood, 1999.
Teaching Literature and Medicine. Ed. Anne Hunsaker Hawkins and Marilyn
   Chandler McEntrye. New York: Modern Language Association, 2000.
The Teacher's Body: Embodiment, Authority, and Identity in the Academy. Ed.
   Diane P. Freedman and Martha Stoddard Holmes. New York: State Univ.
   of New York Press, 2003.

Theodore Deppe

ℰ

Deppe's words lead the reader on an archeological dig of the heart and soul in poems rich with history yet crackling with modernity. Inspired as much by the neighborhood ballpark as by the sea cliffs of the Irish coast, Deppe unites imagination and reality in poems that entertain and enlighten the reader. In his commentary Deppe tells us about the truth of poetry and how the truth gets written. Although he writes easily of the writing process, he prefers to let his poems tell their own stories, and each poem does exactly that as it escorts the reader through its compact and luminous world.

HOW DOES A POEM BEGIN? Often, for me, it starts with surprise: when I encounter something unexpected that challenges what I previously believed, my attention is aroused. A makeshift definition: poetry is an act of attention, composed of words, born of surprise.

Perhaps two of the poems here began when I sat down next to a woman I'd never met before. It was a summer evening, and we were seated in the bleachers above a little league ballpark, watching our children play. Am I only imagining this, or did I really tell her we were in paradise? If so, I supported that claim by tracing the etymology of the English word "paradise" to the Persian original, which denotes a green, enclosed pleasure garden or park. Baseball was my favorite childhood game and—if childhood is ever innocent—the sound of a ball meeting a bat conveys a hint of Eden's bliss.

The woman and I talked a little. I was new to town. Then she leaned over and passed on the rumor that began these poems: the mafia donated the land for the park.

I was filled with questions, confused, oddly exhilarated, troubled, and on the track of a poem. The first draft of "Admission, Children's Unit" stuck pretty closely to the events I've described. The second draft was written after I watched *The Godfather* and was struck by Don Corleone's words in the opening frames. With no hint of irony, he tells an undertaker, "You've found paradise in America."

By the fourth draft, I'd included this woman's claim that the mafia was also behind the sex rings in the city where I worked. That led to three lines in which the narrator thinks about a boy on the children's unit whose mother, a prostitute, had burned him with cigarettes. Later, looking at what I'd written, I realized there was more passion in those three lines than in the rest of the poem, so I followed the road with the most energy and wrote "Admission, Children's Unit" as it appears here.

As Robert Frost says, "Like a piece of ice on a hot stove, the poem must ride on its own melting." I start a poem when some event triggers surprise, wonder, anger, or laughter. I end up wherever the poem takes me. In this case, my son, the mafia, the baseball park, and paradise all disappeared by the seventh draft of the poem, and I ended up exploring an event from the hospital that had been pressing on my imagination.

This little league baseball park—that may or may not have been a gift from the mafia—took on almost mythic significance for me. Because it had disappeared entirely from the finished version of "Admission, Children's Unit," I found myself one day starting a new poem about that ballpark. Oddly, sometime during revision the park disappeared again, leaving me with a poem about an AIDS activist. This happened again and again—I'd return to "the mother lode" about the mafia and my son playing baseball, and I'd end up with a poem that had none of the triggering images but still explored the core question: how do we accommodate ourselves to, or resist, evil?

Recently, I finished a poem called "For Don Corleone in Paradise" centering on the images that began "Admissions, Children's Unit" nearly six years ago. I was a bit superstitious about publishing it since those images had been a stimulus for so many poems.

ADMISSION, CHILDREN'S UNIT

Like the story of St. Lawrence that repelled me
when I heard it in high school, how he taught
his disciples to recognize the smell
of sin, then sent them in pairs through the Roman Empire,
separating good from evil, brother from brother.
Scrap of legend I'd forgotten until, interviewing a woman
I drew my breath in and smelled
her, catching a scent that was there, then not there.

She said her son set fire to his own room,
she'd found him fanning it with a comic, and what
should she have done? Her red hair
was pulled back in a braid, she tugged at its flames,
and what she'd done, it turns out, was hold her son
so her boyfriend could burn him with cigarettes.
The details didn't, of course, come out at first,
but I sensed them. The boy's refusal to take off his shirt.
His letting me, finally, lift it to his shoulders
and examine the six wounds, raised, ashy, second
or third degree, arranged in a cross.

Silence in the room, and then the mother blaming
the boyfriend, blaming the boy himself.
I kept talking to her in a calm voice, straining
for something I thought I smelled beneath
her cheap perfume, a scent—how can I describe this?—
as if something not physical had begun to rot.

I'd like to say all this happened when I first started
to work as a nurse, before I'd learned not to judge
the parents, but this was last week, the mother was crying,
I thought of handing her a box of tissues, and didn't.

When the Romans crucified Lawrence,
he asked Jesus to forgive him for judging others.
He wept on the cross because he smelled his own sin.

Sullen and wordless, the boy got up, brought his mother
the scented, blue Kleenex from my desk,
pressed his head into her side. Bunching
the bottom of her sweatshirt in both hands,
he anchored himself to her. Glared at me.
It took four of us to pry him from his mother's arms.

For Don Corleone in Paradise

All day darkness slams the kitchen windows
   as we bake and clean for Thanksgiving.

Wind snaps branches, severs shingles, impresses on us
    its ability to obliterate—
        with a few notchings-up of the blast—
  everything.
From a pay phone our son calls:
  four hours on the road
  and Michael's hardly closer
      to our new home than when he set out.
Bad enough the roads are packed and stormy, but
  an hour ago, lost outside Worcester,
    he was snared in a roadblock
  as police searched car-to-car for drive-by killers.
    Flashlights probed
        the cluttered interior of Michael's car
studied him closely, rain pelting his shoulder-length hair:
  the more he tried to appear innocent
the more he felt unfathomably guilty.
    Finally, the face in the orange parka
      gave directions Michael couldn't remember
once the flashlight waved him on.

        Here, at least, the cooking's done
  so I turn on the radio as I wash up, listen
    to accounts of the gangland slaying.
Last month, I watched *The Godfather* and recall now its opening:
    voice-over-darkness: *I believe*
in America. The screen's still dark
    so your first time viewing the movie
you don't know this credo's
      spoken by an undertaker.

Sidelit, Brando appears, acknowledges,
    You've found paradise in America.
Paradise: from the Persian word for enclosed park
  or pleasure garden. And I'm back one more time to this:
my children learned baseball in a park donated to our town
    by the Mafia.
      I watched ten-year-old Michael
shield his eyes with his glove, divide

his attention between his game and
　　the light-struck gulls that ghosted down
　　　　to squabble over peanuts in left field.
　Late sun battered his uniform to a glow I want
　　　　　to call innocence.
None of us in that town, though, were very innocent –
　　we all knew, or thought we knew;
but lacking proof
　　we could keep quiet. And those we'd like to call evil
　　　doted on us:
　　the foundation that fronted the mob
　　　gave us our fire station as well as the ballpark.

At last, Michael arrives and we gather beneath
　　a ring of candles while the gale shakes our windows.
My wife quotes Paul Durcan, *The set table*
　　which is the city of God, a phrase I love,
　　but why do I keep thinking of that gift of a ballpark?
　　　Across the table, in his Grateful Dead T-shirt,
Michael is shyly telling jokes
　　and I'm sure, suddenly, it's the same shirt he wore
　　　　when he shoved past me
　　how many years ago
in argument: I pinned him to the floor and he slipped
　　a fist loose and bloodied my nose, startling us both.
Struggling to our feet, we didn't know
　　whether to flail at each other or embrace
　　and take stock. It was, at least,
the only time we laid a hand on each other in anger.

　Last year I worked the adolescent unit
　　and presided over a Thanksgiving dinner
for gang members and would-be suicides.
　　　Rochelle, fourteen, wanted each of us
　　to name something we were grateful for, and, surprise,
the kids were eager to affirm what they could.
　　　We took turns until Damion stood up to say,
　I am not thankful for my father
　　　who offed himself in our kitchen,

and I am not thankful for my mom who tried to teach me
    not to steal
        by holding my hands in boiling water.
But I do give thanks for my brothers in the Latin Kings,
    the only family who will back me—he gripped
        the table as he spoke as if he'd like to fling
        the feast across the room—*no matter what you assholes*
try to do to me.

                I was able, somehow,
to talk him to his room where the two of us shared
    our holiday meal at his bedside table
and spoke of family. I recall how earnestly
        he said the word, *family*,
    and how double-edged it rang. I don't know how
            to say the word properly—
no family is innocent—but if I could pronounce it correctly
    it would sound like that paradise from which
we've all been banished, that home we can never find alone.

For a long time I was troubled by a disconnection in my life. I worked with clients who suffered, and then I drove home and tried to unwind and enjoy myself. I kept thinking of Anton Chekhov's short story, "Gooseberries," which meditates powerfully on the way we can only be happy when we forget that others are suffering. I wanted to find a way to live happily without, at the same time, ignoring those who were in torment.

Writing turned out to be one way to bridge those aspects of my life. I had for years resisted writing about my hospital experiences, not wanting to use some tragic event to get a good poem. Along with ethical considerations, there were issues of confidentiality. "Admission, Children's Unit" provided a breakthrough. I found myself inventing things that I hoped were nonetheless true. Having worked with many abused children, I was able to create a parafactual situation. Drawing on those experiences, I "made up" something I hope is emotionally true. As Picasso said, "Art is the lie that tells the truth."

This process of making up characters through composites is well known to fiction writers but seems less common to poets. It's a useful strategy for the nurse who wants to write about clients.

My mother-in-law knew how I worked and sometimes asked me to talk about a given poem's background. I've dedicated "The Japanese Deer" to her.

THE JAPANESE DEER

*For Denny Lynn, who likes to know what's true in my poems
and what's "made up."*

What's true in this is that Luis, not his real name,
sat next to me on the field trip to the Lost Village
because I didn't trust him farther back in the van.
Also true, when we returned to the Children's Unit,
he drew me a picture with scented markers
in which rabbit-sized deer leapt through a dangling fence
while a funnel cloud labeled "Hurricane Gloria"
shot apple blossoms through the air.

Luis didn't, however, see the Japanese deer
though I'd told him to watch for twelve-point bucks
the size of fawns. Years ago, before they were loosed
by Gloria, I sometimes fed that herd
at Henry Joy's deer yard, a few miles
from the Lost Village's unmarked logging road.
Hard to say if they still survive in those hills,
tame, miniature deer that ate from the hands of strangers.

I told the kids I'd never been to the Lost Village.
Not true. I think I wanted them to believe
we might get lost finding it, might have to get lost,
unnecessary pretence since I led them
unintentionally down a wrong path,
had to double back, follow a cut to a stream
where gold finches flashed their dull fire
beside the ruins of a mill.

Further back, cellar holes like sunken gardens,
foundations reclaimed by blackberries and ferns.
No historical marker here,
only a friend's story of an English deserter
who fled to the wilds of Connecticut
and fathered sixteen children, some lodged now
beneath fiddleheads, the low cemetery walls
unable to hold back the forest.

But what surprised me that day
was the apparition of apple blossoms
seen through the woods, children breaking ranks
and running. I tried to judge the danger:
wind whipped the sweet, heavy scent
of flowers about the orchard, children rode
the lower branches, while dead limbs
creaked in trees unpruned a hundred years.

What's true in this story is that Marisol,
raped repeatedly by her mother's boyfriend,
and Luis, who watched from the hall as his stepfather
stabbed his mother to death—nothing
can change those facts—climbed for a short time
above the brambled understory, outside history,
discovered a fragrant scent on their hands,
shredded more petals, rubbed the smell deep in their skin.

As I drove back-roads to the hospital
a few of the girls slept,
apple sprays wilting in their hair.
A white-tailed doe looked up
from the center of the asphalt, froze,
then bounded into the evening woods
before most of the children saw her.
Back on the unit, though, they were sure

they'd seen one of the Japanese deer—
some had seen the whole herd, small as fawns,
watching silently from the shadows.
Now, on my study wall, the drawing Luis gave me:
deer he never saw leap in pairs
through an autumn storm that kicks up
spring flowers, impossible, all of it,
but this is the way he remembers it; this is the truth.

Nurses don't get sabbaticals, so after twenty years of getting up early to write, then spending my lunch breaks working on poems, I reached a point where the writing needed to be given my full efforts. Meanwhile, the hospital job

I had enjoyed for many years had become unrecognizable: trying to survive in an era of managed care, the hospital moved adolescent patients onto the same unit as the small children I'd cared for, and the new double unit felt untherapeutic. Unable to change the situation, I decided it was time to leave and write full time.

Happily, my wife agreed. We gave notice to our employers, sold our house, and rented the southernmost house in Ireland. On Cape Clear Island, eight miles off the coast of County Cork, we had dramatic sea cliffs for a backyard and plenty of gales to keep us inside writing.

Our plan was to go to Ireland for a year and then return to the United States and find a new job, perhaps in community health. At the end of the year, however, I was offered a job teaching poetry in a graduate program in Donegal. For a year and a half I served as writer-in-residence there, and then an NEA grant made it possible to return to Cape Clear for some more full-time writing.

I haven't forgotten the children I cared for in the hospital. Just as I once found their stories pressing on my imagination while I tried to write about a little league baseball field, now they reappeared time and again in poems set in Ireland.

Recently, we returned to the United States so I could take a job as writer-in-residence in Andover, Massachusetts. However, I keep my nursing license up to date and imagine I will one day return to work as an RN.

Love in dreams, Dostoyevsky wrote, is easy. However, he termed love in action "a harsh and dreadful thing." My years of nursing called forth much of the best in me. It was a period in which the various parts of my life felt integrated. Art and work and prayer and love were woven together into something important.

Do I second-guess my decision to write and teach instead of caring for clients? Sometimes. But as Chaim Potok's young painter Asher Lev learned, there will always be guilt. The artist must allow that guilt to help create the art.

MARISOL

When I quit my nursing job
to write in Ireland,
I stepped out into summer stars

and clicked my heels in the air.
Security cameras
caught my leap

and the supervisor
froze the frame all night
so day shift could see
that look of pure joy.

Strange now, to think
Marisol had just been readmitted.

Did Dante feel guilty
as he left the inferno?—all those voices calling,
remember us to the living—

I can be watching the island children
run down the pier after a field trip
to the mainland, or a hooded crow
might crack a mollusk on the rocks, and—

Beautiful Marisol.
Her pale, dirty face framed
by matted black hair.

Some keenness behind those dark eyes
as if she'd been raised by wolves.
Marisol, who'd stabbed her foster father
with a pencil: her fourth failed placement.

Marisol, who'd first
come to our children's unit
when she was five—something broken
behind those eyes, and fierce—

At the seawall, the island children call
to the spring tide to swell up
and pelt them
with rocks and spray.

They shriek, cover their heads and run,
then return laughing to the slipway
and taunt the sea again.

And the children in the hospital courtyard?
Those who will call out to anyone
beyond the high, link fence?
Want to or not, I see them:

Marisol strides on low stilts
through the locked garden
and won't look at her birthmother

who's finally come to visit.
She plants one leg down and
swings her hip into the next step:

her mother and that nurse
can go to hell
till this dance is played out,

back straight, head high,
everyone calling.

The speaker of the poem "The Funeral March of Adolf Wölfli" is not Ted Deppe but the nurse Lisa Becker who once took care of the schizophrenic painter, musician, poet, and inventor Adolf Wölfli. Taking on the persona of a Swiss nurse allowed me to speak about issues that were important to me while transcending the merely personal.

The Polish writer Adam Zagajewski calls form and chaos "the twin angels of art."

Every poem needs to find some sort of form, whether it is composed using traditional structures like the sonnet or written in free verse. But it also needs to let in a little chaos, something unexpected, if it is to become truly alive. It needs to allow in surprise and go beyond what we could predict or plan.

Adolf Wölfli suffered from hallucinations; his life was filled with chaos. But he imposed what measure and meaning he could on that difficult inner life, and the results are startling works of what is now called Outsider Art. Without any formal training, he made up his own rules.

A typical Wölfli painting includes dense musical scores. These notes might disappear into train tunnels guarded by angels and then reappear in another part of his native city, Bern. No one could decipher Wölfli's musical system, and for years art critics felt the notes were merely decorative. Recently, experts

have broken the code and his music has been performed for the first time. I
hope someday to hear it.

THE FUNERAL MARCH OF ADOLF WÖLFLI

From the oral history of Lisa Becker taken in
Bern, Switzerland, 1970.

I found that art would keep him quiet. After breaking
a fellow patient's wrist, he was isolated for years

—I brought him colored pencils and newsprint
and he drew all day, or composed music in a system

God revealed to him. For a time he thought he loved me.
For a time my face appeared in every drawing he made.

He wrote the "Santa Lisa Polka" for me, hardly danceable, but—
despite the homemade paper trumpet he hummed on—

haunting, and mine. He said, once, if I married him,
he'd abdicate his kingdom, write a waltz for me each day.

Strange, then, after he died, to search in vain
through his eight-thousand-page *Funeral March*, looking

for something—anything—I could play before we buried him.
His masterpiece reached to the ceiling of his cell,

hand-sewn scores in which the music constantly gave way
to drawings or ads from magazines. What might have been

eighth notes floated above maps or rambling prayers,
and then staves appeared with no notes at all—

this was the work he'd curse me for disturbing!
The night before his funeral, I sorted through

those composition books and found no sustained melody—
but what did I expect? When he worked, he had a ritual

of rolling up his shirt sleeves and trousers
that took hours, interrupted by his voices. He'd start

drawing in the margins and press inward, filling each space,
singing to himself like a boy. Oh, he was more selfish

than a child, incapable of loving anyone. I never told him
I wasn't married. I took care of him thirty years, longer

than most marriages last! Such a strange, ugly fellow—
our yellow-fingered, warp-nailed, one-man Renaissance.

He'd consume his week's supply of pencils in three days,
then beg for more—against the doctor's orders I gave them.

His *March* was signed, "St. Adolf, Chief Music Director,
Painter, Writer, Inventor of 160 Highly Valuable Inventions,

Victor of Mammoth Battles, Giant-Theatre-Director,
Great God, Mental Patient, Casualty."

In some ways I was relieved when he died, as if a blizzard
finally howled away and I could start to shovel out.

He didn't want to leave a few perfect works behind him.
He wanted to lift up everything, wanted to give

the whole dying world lasting form.
There were lucid moments when he knew he was mad—

he could almost imagine what a normal life might be.
I'd go home and practice piano every night.

I'd play Beethoven, feel the moments things caught fire,
but couldn't myself become flame.

Page upon page of his *March*, containing, he said, everything
and everyone he'd ever loved, and not a single tune

I could play for his funeral. Not even the "Santa Lisa Polka."
We buried him without music. There is nothing

I blame myself for more. We buried him without music
and for two weeks I took to bed. Then one night—

it was snowing—I rolled up the sleeves of my nightdress.
I pinned up the hem, then puzzled over a line of music

that vanished in a field of painted irises, purple flags
instead of notes waving under a sky of sharps and flats.

I closed my eyes and began to play. I didn't know
what my hands were doing. Snow kept falling,

silences tumbled forward, winged notes soared
above chipped ivory keys. I played what I could

of his *Funeral March*—imperfectly, of course,
only in fragments—I played the *Funeral March*

of Adolf Wölfli, everything dark, falling, silver.

In nursing school, I was taught that nursing was a science. There's a case to be
made for that, but I have always felt that nursing is an art that juggles many
sciences. Both nursing and poetry are ways of practicing the art of attention.
Attention, I believe, is almost the same thing as love. What we pay attention
to is what we truly care about. Call nursing the art of caring, if you like, or the
art of putting love in action.

Poetry Publications

Deppe's poetry publications include the following books:

Cape Clear: New and Selected Poems. Cliffs of Moher, Ireland: Salmon Poetry,
  2002.
Children of the Air. Farmington, Maine: Alice James Books, 1990.
Necessary Journeys. Chapbook. Hartford, Conn.: Andrew Mountain Books,
  1988.
The Wanderer King. Farmington, Maine: Alice James Books, 1996.

Deppe has poems published in the following journals:

Boulevard; Harper's Magazine; Kenyon Review; New England Review; Plough-shares; Poetry; Poetry Ireland Review; Prairie Schooner; Southern Review.

Deppe's poetry is included in the following anthologies:

Between the Heartbeats: Poetry and Prose by Nurses. Ed. Cortney Davis and Judy Schaefer. Iowa City: Univ. of Iowa Press, 1995.

Intensive Care: More Poetry and Prose by Nurses. Ed. Cortney Davis and Judy Schaefer. Iowa City: Univ. of Iowa Press, 2003.

A Life In Medicine: A Literary Anthology. Ed. Robert Coles and Randy Testa. New York: New Press, 2002.

The Pushcart Prize 2000: Best of the Small Presses. Ed. Bill Henderson. Wainscott, N.Y.: Pushcart Press, 2000.

Three Genres: The Writing of Poetry, Fiction, and Drama. Ed. Stephen Minot. Upper Saddle River, N.J.: Prentice Hall, 2002.

Sandra Bishop Ebner

જ&

Like most of the nurse-poets in this book, Ebner started writing as a child, long before she was a nurse. Early on she learned the transforming power of language. Poems, like nursing tasks, are acts of transformation. Poems are healing, especially for the poet, and Ebner tells us that her poetry is the creation of a place of temporary detachment and, subsequently, a space for rest and reparation. Her poems are inspired by simple pleasures such as movement in a car or by onerous tasks such as filling out a daily activity log. She candidly invites us into her interior world of poetry making and we see firsthand how her poetry works for her—and for us—to our delight.

WHEN I WAS A CHILD of eight, I was faced with an inexplicable dilemma. On the one hand I wanted desperately for my father to come out of the bar and take me home. I knew that he would be more congenial than usual—attentive, even. I sat in the back of his '50s Chevy for longer than it takes the sun to go down behind the west end of the village green, bouncing up and down, trying not to pee on the seat. On the other hand, when my father finally did come out to the car, I knew the drive home could be erratic enough to take my life.

I suspect there is a lot of buried emotion behind that story, and the poem "My Father's Violin" is one of my favorites, partly because of the circumstances behind the crafting of that poem. I wrote the poem years ago, and it taught me that I could craft a poem with detachment—without the emotion attached to the speaker's situation (or the writer's situation), which was behind the writing of many of my other poems. This time, the emotional nudge wasn't there. I decided to use the names of different parts of the violin as a means of setting up a condition—a child's world in which the speaker, the child, longs for a relationship with the unavailable father. Hopefully what results from the work—what touches a chord of memory in the reader—is the truth of the poem, not necessarily my original thought and not necessarily the facts, but the "something else" that is achieved by the crafting of the poem.

MY FATHER'S VIOLIN

If I could have been the bow in your hand,
the horsehair sliding over the fingerboard,
the music resonating from the soundpost,
the dust on the sidewall/rib,
the chin rest.

If I could have been a tuning peg,
or the peg box,
or the empty spaces of the F-shaped holes
your fingers touched,
the wood grain.

I would have been anything. And you
never noticed how I waited in the stairwell.
how I leaned against the wall
listening

to the music. Startled by the sound
of the violin dropping hard on the floor.
Replaced by the booze in your brain.

I would never say anything.
Silent, like the strings
on your violin I hold,
then close up cold in its case.

I got a phone call from Leo Connellan, once Connecticut's poet laureate, after he finished reading my manuscript. He congratulated me on what he thought were some very significant poems. Weeks later, when I told him I had decided not to publish many of them (those I suspected would hurt some family members), he flipped. He was so angry with me. "Your children are grown. They don't need protecting," he spit out. He tried his best to convince me that what was important was the work, not anyone's response to the work.

I can always publish the poems, I reminded myself, but I can never unpublish them. "My Father's Violin" is not one that I considered excluding, but even that poem touched a chord of sorrow in my mother.

I like the "show, don't tell" aspect of the poem "Size 8 Surgical Gloves," and the raw anger in the poem. This time, I was not detached from the anger, not necessarily warranted, that I felt at this particular point in time toward a physician. That I could transform my anger into a poem was fun and cathartic, to say the least.

SIZE 8 SURGICAL GLOVES

I have anger.
I can smell it.
Rancid odor no
deodorant can hide

rises from my armpits.
They itch and the stench
sticks to my fingertips.
I could kill.

Take a surgery-sharp knife,
make a clean-cut incision
from the xiphoid process
to the symphysis pubis,

spread skin apart.
Watch how the tip of the heart
stops moving.

Examine particles of undigested
food where the stomach is.
Listen to the scream

of saw

as it splits sternum.

Hold smooth, serous
coated spleen with latex-gloved
hand, gently squeeze.

I would fill the bladder with just
enough helium to set it afloat
to the sky

then hand feed bite-size
pieces of warm liver
to well-fed cats.

Nursing poems are, in some ways, more difficult to write. How does one write about one's work when one has the moral and legal obligation to keep the conditions and experiences of patients confidential? The "facts" need to be "fictionalized," which, in actuality, is often true in most poems or works of art when imagination goes to work. So many lives are similar in so many ways, and as much as I create and invent the conditions and the characters within the poems, they are still based on a variety of experience that I would not be exposed to if, indeed, I were not a visiting nurse going into the homes of those in need of my care. Thus, while the characters in the poems are based on situations and human conditions that exist on some level, genders change, family compositions change, and medical conditions change. Imagination, the integral part of any poem, reflects, I think, what is already contained in memory in perhaps an unformed way. I use my imagination to conjure up ideas about death or love or betrayal, for example, and then use language to create the work. Maybe, if I'm original and lucky, I've created something (usually something other than what it started out to be) called a poem. I am always reluctant to interpret or "believe" my poems as they begin to come into form. What I'm writing—what a speaker is saying—is rarely what is being "said." The use and work of imagination is particularly important when creating poems based on professional work experience. I use my imagination, which is sparked by what I see, feel, remember, and even forget, then revise or recreate all that in a poem. I create and manipulate the facts—the inspiration.

"Daily Activity Log" is an ultimate expression of a truth, insofar as it reveals a nurse's long day of interventions—possibly empathic, possibly not—with regard to a variety of mental health conditions. The loneliness in that—the visit, the emotional holding by the nurse, the energy required, and lastly the ultimate filling out of a time sheet—what the bosses, the administrators, get to "see." What is *truly* significant is what administration is "blind" to, and the sad juxtaposition of that. Another "truth" in the poem, or a next poem, possibly, is that the nurse is also on the wellness/illness continuum along with all human beings. The question often hovering in that invisible space is whether the patient is a mirror for the caregiver's own self.

DAILY ACTIVITY LOG

1st visit
She's lying on urine-
    soaked sheets—whiskey
  bottle empty on the floor.
I say her name,
wrap the cuff around a flab
    of arm, can almost detect
      an 80 over 40, tachycardia, eyes roll. She groans—
two EMTS (I've dialed 911)
lift her; the sound

of sirens disappears as she's taken up the hill . . .

2nd
I say to him,
You missed three mornings' meds
and all your bedtime pills are still there.
They're fucking with my mind. He sucks cigarette smoke,
blows out, throws the medication cassette—
Valproic Acid, Cogentin, Clonazepam
  scatter in a pattern on the floor . . .
3rd
6.7 miles later the patient tells me
someone put two hundred dollars
    in her drawer to buy
the dog, but the old man next door keeps
sneaking into her house—
must be at night, but the doors
        are locked—maybe he comes in through the window . . .
4th
Quick Haldol injection next, parkinsonism
worse
than his beautiful, in their metaphoric glory, delusions.
He starts to walk,
starts to walk, starts to walk again . . .
5th
What would you do in an emergency
if you needed someone immediately?

Well I . . . she stares at the phone, frowns . . . *I would,*
would would, and put this?
  pick this, this up? the number
    on the handset a jumbled connection to somewhere
where   she knew   at one time
she had known   what to do,   and the dog
piss and shit collect on the floor
there's a black crust
on the bottom of the pot she had
    forgotten again to turn off the stove . . .
6th
Grandiosity gone in the next patient,
there, in a shamble
      of house where the roof leaks and the eaves
  are filled with leaves.

Her face, bruised—What happened to you?
I tried to call the police,
he kept, kept slamming the phone
      down. I can't move my goddamned arm.
Her spouse, now in his drunken sleep upstairs, had dragged
  her into the kitchen.
You can call the police now, if you want to.
And when they take him away,
the way he looks at me I know he wants to kill me . . .

Employee name. Title. Company Branch.
Odometer start. Odometer end. Time in.
Time out. Total number of miles traveled.
Total amount of time spent in the home.

I remember the first time I experienced music in rhyme, even before I knew
the words "poem" and "rhyme" existed. I came across the lines "Blessings
on this little man, / barefoot boy with cheeks of tan. / With thine upturned
pantaloons, / and thy merry whistled tunes. / With thy red lip redder still, /
kissed by strawberries on the hill." I still remember the sense of surprise and
delight I felt with the sound of those lines from "The Barefoot Boy," written
by John Greenleaf Whittier in 1855.

  I started writing poetry at age nine. I was shy and did not show my poems
to anyone, especially not to teachers, one of whom had accused me (in front

of my classmates) of lifting what were my own words to write a black stallion story when I was in seventh grade. I'd written it during recess, and fortunately another teacher, who had allowed me to stay in because I had not done my homework, verified that I had written it. I had a similar experience as a freshman in high school. It was another prose piece and, like the black stallion piece, written quickly. This time, the teacher tried to test me by telling me to write it again from memory. I was able to, and she actually seemed disappointed. No apology from her, but I was older and a little braver and purposely started handing in poems filled with drunken family images. She returned them, saying, in effect, that she was tired of getting my inappropriate and depressing poems.

But as a nine-year-old, I was making rhyming poems. Writing gave me what I sensed I didn't have at the time: a voice, and—words to communicate with my shy self. Years later, I realized that women continue to struggle with articulating in a language that is primarily patriarchal, but that's a whole different territory. At that young age, I could put things down on paper and the words would speak back to me. Long before I realized that poems are like dreams—they teach us what we didn't know we already knew—I was learning from my writing. I was beginning to define myself and my surroundings, to make some sense of things. Like most writers, the motivation came out of the need to use language to define and recreate.

As a child, I read mostly prose. My oldest sister gave me Nancy Drew and Hardy Boys mysteries to read and I was hooked. I didn't start reading poetry with any seriousness until high school. I fell in love with twentieth-century American poet Edna St. Vincent Millay's writing. I memorized "Renascence," all 214 lines. I was fortunate to have an English teacher who introduced us to some well-known English and American poets. She was also the first teacher who gave me positive feedback on and encouraged my writing. Often, teachers do not realize how damaging or inspiring they can be—what effect they have on a young mind.

I wrote some fairly decent sonnets and odes, none of which I saved, but I have committed to memory two of my nine-year-old rhyming poems. I felt a sense of delight when I realized I had written my first poem ever. I loved that I was able to make end words rhyme—the only kind of poem I thought existed. The child in the poem (now the adult interpreting it!) had a life punctuated by family difficulties, made worse by a larger culture that, in essence, insisted that preadolescent girls dissociate from who they really are in order to fit into a society that subtly and not so subtly demanded that they be quiet, be nice, be ladylike, defer to boys, bounce the basketball only three times in a row, and so forth. So I think the child in the poem longed to fly away from all of that, without, of course, an understanding of what "all of that" was, in order to have some semblance of control, in order to be free. I was also a rather pragmatic child, and was able to incorporate a certain sense of acceptance into what I was able to do.

Did I understand the transforming power of art at the time—that in creating the work, I was experiencing, on some level, the freedom I longed for? Not in any intellectual manner, but I started writing poems and, even if in secret, started creating, transforming, and taking control of things.

IF I COULD FLY

One day I lifted my head up high,
and as I looked up at the sky,
I wondered how nice it would be
if I could really fly.
If I could drift up with the breeze
and maybe rest on limbs of trees,
oh, how happy I would be.
But then I thought as I looked back down
how lucky I really am.
To be able to walk upon the ground
and on the soft smooth sand.
To be able to run and jump with glee.
I think I'll let the birds fly for me.

I went through a religious period, which intensified in high school, a probable reaction, in part, to developing a crush on the new, young assistant parish priest. I memorized lines from Francis Thompson's "The Hound of Heaven" and delved into the writings of St. John of the Cross and St. Theresa of Avila, who founded the Discalced Carmelite Nuns. I started going to daily mass. I'd kneel before the statue of St. Theresa of the Roses and think, How safe a life like that would be!

I entered a Carmelite Monastery. The whole town, practically, gave me a going-away testimonial. The cloistered experience was, on one hand, beautiful, and, on the other, utterly strange. Fortunately, I maintained a sense of humor throughout most of the time I spent enclosed and out of touch with society, and I kept a journal. In retrospect, the journal writing was what kept me focused and sane. "Someday, Sister Sandra, you'll be buried here," Sister Mary of the Trinity said to me as we made our daily walk past some grave stones within the walls of the monastery. I fled in less than six months.

I started redating the boy from high school. His aunt, who was a visiting nurse, suggested I become an LPN. I did that, got married, had three children, and became a not-so-modern "nonworking" housewife and mother.

I went back for an associate's degree in nursing when the children were in school. I discovered twentieth-century American poet Anne Sexton in college. My writing style had long since moved away from rhyme. Reading Anne Sexton influenced me greatly. I had already read poets such as nineteenth-century American poet Emily Dickinson and twentieth-century American poet Elizabeth Bishop, but I identified with Sexton. Her work seemed to give me the courage to start writing what I suppose could be called confessional poems, although I believe that term is a misnomer. Sexton apparently began a poem with a phrase or an idea and then felt a sudden interruption of her whole life—a call to action, a call to write a poem. What poet can't identify with that? I still have *The New York Times* October 6, 1974, obituary announcing her probable suicide.

During my married years and while writing on a regular basis, I met Helen Trubek Glenn at a cocktail party. We clicked—we were both nurses and we both wrote poetry. She was interested in starting a women's poetry group and asked me to join. I had gotten some wonderful feedback and encouragement from a college English professor, but for the most part I still didn't share my poems, so I was pretty nervous just before our first meeting. We were to talk a bit about ourselves and read a poem or two. We started conversing with one another before everyone sat down. I made a quick exit to the bathroom and thought about leaving then and there. I stayed enclosed for several minutes, convincing myself to stay. My turn came. The other women liked my work. I could tell.

Since then, those monthly meetings have become a place to read poems, have them witnessed, and find supportive and constructive criticism. And we are truthful. The regular feedback and experience critiquing helps tremendously with the craft and provides motivation to write new poems.

My nursing experience was on a medical surgical floor, a bit in maternity, ICU, and then eight years in the dialysis unit—I became the home peritoneal dialysis nurse instructor. My first nursing love, however, had always been in the field of mental health. During my psychiatric rotation in school, one of my instructors recommended that specialty to me. She said I had an intuitive sense in my approach to patients that went beyond the theoretical knowledge base. I seemed to be very good at developing a rapport and responding to intense situations with calm and dignity. Before I "knew" theoretically what I was doing, I could put "the whammy" on a confused elderly woman trying to flee her hospital room in the middle on the night, hold her hand, and say, "It's OK now. Here, get some sleep. I'll sit with you."

I made the decision to get a good medical surgical background first; however, after years of hospital nursing, I finally entered the world of psychiatric nursing. I worked in a dual-diagnosis residential setting, and then went on to psychiatric case management for a visiting-nurse service. I had also gone back to school. The home-environment perspective is extraordinary and, obviously, unlike any other. Intuition and empathy depend upon one's self-awareness, but one must know what it's like to sit in the other chair. I believe that therapy is an important and necessary way to acquire some sense of self-knowledge (writing can do that too, to an extent) and I needed to revise some of my own life, so I started the long, hard road toward self-awareness.

My writing flourished during those years. I took some workshops with poets like Sharon Olds, whose work I came to admire. I went on some "Women, Wilderness, Writing Retreats." I also went "public," so to speak, and started reading at open-mic events. I began to enjoy the audience response.

I had the dubious distinction of ending up on the 1994 Connecticut Poetry Slam Team. It was marvelous. The nationals were in Asheville, North Carolina. What a hoopla event that was, and I got to perform in front of hundreds of people "Silent Night/Holy Night," a poem about using a chain saw inside the house (after the divorce) in an attempt to pare down the trunk of a Christmas tree so I could fit it into the stand. Slam poetry is in-your-face-performance poetry and different from what I was writing.

Most of my poems are other than nursing poems. There is a connection, however, between my work and my writing. Not because I am necessarily writing about the work, but because creating—doing the art—is healing. And of course, there is the creative side to dealing with illness in general, mental illness in particular. I think the fact that I am a poet—and it took me a long time to call myself "a poet"—informs my nursing, to a degree. Maybe as poets we do "see" things a little differently. I listen to what's behind what is said. I recognize some amazing metaphors in the delusional thinking of patients with the clinical label of paranoid schizophrenia, for example. We live in a crazy world. I have seen an interesting poemlike nature in much of the delusional thinking that attempts to keep that craziness at bay.

During the period of time that I was working forty hours a week, and well aware of the vicarious post-traumatic stress that caregivers are vulnerable to, especially if they are good at what they do, I was aware, also, of how writing, reading, and being "a poet" helped to relieve much of that stress. We provide an emotional holding environment for patients. That takes tremendous energy. The work of writing, of engaging in one's art form—can be a way of resting.

THE CURE

Night hovers.
Window shades up.
Cassiopeia resembles nothing
more than one letter
of light
too far away
to wish on.
Bones tired of holding
flesh together.
She has decided to go
to sleep.
The long black sleep
of the soul wanting
to forget how the body feels
to be split mid-chest.
She has made clean slits.
Each artery, each wrist,
and the bed is a warm,
red well.
She noticed the moon
last.
Tonight it's a sliver.
Harmless as a fingernail.

In "The Cure," the image of the moon's fingernail shape, distant and harm-less, is one that I had written several years ago in a prose piece. It ended up being the only line I liked—I discarded the prose piece and kept the line. I wanted to use it, but forcing lines into a poem usually feels like that: forced. The poem started to come into form, and I had the feeling that I wanted the sliver of moon to be the last thing seen by the someone in the poem. The poem became a death poem and an exercise, of sorts, to keep it as spare as the moon image as possible.

Poetry is more like the visual arts than we sometimes think. For example, I can create the words on the page, or I can create the negative space around those words. I was attempting to do that. I also decided I wanted the moon image to be seen "last" by the reader; I wanted the sense of time to extend beyond "her" death, and I wanted the reader to be in that time, to feel it. I sent it to *The Comstock Review's* annual poetry contest. Mary Oliver, that year's judge, gave it a special merit. That acknowledgement felt good, but there were still some things about the poem I didn't like. Short poems need particularly strong closing lines, and my closing lines needed improvement. There were also a couple of words the poem didn't need, and I pared it down even more.

AUTOPSY NO. 24722

Dead February 4th. He was sixty-five. That's young, isn't it?
Patient with a ten-year history
of intermittent claudication, documented
inferior wall myocardial infarction.
A photograph shows him young. So handsome.
He would pour black molasses on his plate,
soak it up with bread, joke about
what he might run out of first, molasses
or bread; if molasses, add molasses, if bread, bread.
No way to end, he'd grin.

The right coronary artery almost
completely occluded one centimeter from its origin.
Yesterday morning, snow until midnight. Can each flake
be different? Clumps fall from pines—their branches
laden, lift again to tree shape.

The LAD 90% stenosed two centimeters from the bifurcation.
The circumflex contains numerous plaques.
The cat eyes me from outside the window.
What does its longing feel like?
What will my children remember of me?
How thin the skin that covers my veins.
Catheterization revealed almost complete
occlusion of right coronary.
My mother walks from the alter.
Host dissolving on her tongue, she drops to her knees,
a prayer position, heavy head lowered to her arms,
my father surrounded by flowers.
Contrast material fills the vein
in a retrograde manner
from the left coronary. Little filling seen
distal to anastomosis.

Where is the space between children
and their grief?
How else do the dead resurrect themselves?
Myocardial fibrosis—extensive.
My mother's sobbing is the finest offering,
better than Hail Marys, better than the whole rosary—
a novena—her no-words shaking, and the lost husband
will not know the holiness of this sorrow.
I am afraid to touch her
before I kneel down to her. Hold her.

I found my father's autopsy report in a file drawer during some cleaning-out of things. I had read the autopsy years before, but reading it again, I was struck by how distant and cold this clinical language is, and I began to wonder about the pathologist who performed the autopsy. How detached from all emotion. That's not a criticism. One would have to be detached, but what I wanted to do was to add some humanity to the experience of it. I could do this by writing, and I needed to write something. I also found some of the clinical language to be exquisite, and decided to use the technical autopsy language for some of the lines, juxtaposed with personal, anecdotal, human-condition language. I wrote draft after draft, originally four pages. I put it away. Took it out. Kept chiseling away at it.

In 1998 I was approached by a publisher with the request to publish a book of my poems. I was both flattered and surprised. It is difficult to get a manuscript published, and much more accomplished poets than I have not been published. I had never sent in a manuscript. I had never even compiled one to send. I went home that evening and started to look through my work. I'll have to write all new poems, I thought. Nothing is acceptable. Talk about poor sleep patterns that night.

The next morning I called my friend Leo. I had met Leo Connellan before he became Connecticut's poet laureate. We were friends. He would call me on a regular basis. Sometimes I would have to slip into a therapeutic mode, and anyone who knew and loved the late Leo Connellan knows what I'm talking about. Our roles reversed that day. His counsel was wonderfully reassuring. "I do not compare myself to other poets. I am no Seamus Heaney, nor am I a T. S. Eliot. I am Leo Connellan. I write the best that I can write, and that is the best that I can do." Leo did not mean that we should not strive to write better. He was telling me to embrace my own style, embrace who I am. I spent the day doing that—embracing what were my best poems—and in doing so, I was embracing myself.

My daughter, who is a visual artist, agreed to design the cover. Her art has an extraordinary order to it—contemporary pieces evocative of landscapes that often "do" what I try to "do" in my writing. That collaboration alone was an amazing and tender experience. The book's title was chosen from several possible ideas, but *The Space Between* refers to a phenomenon I have been interested in and witness to for years. The observation of that third thing that exists between two people, between a person and experience. That invisible energy that comes into being and hovers there.

Recently, I started going through notebooks and journals and I am realizing again how I can catch the poetic moments. I can catch those images of inspiration almost the way my father could catch fish with string and worms, up in the Allagash, along the St. John River in Maine.

Several years ago, I drove from Dayton, Ohio, to Cleveland. The glory and detail of the landscape as I moved toward and then past it created my own hallucination—optical illusions. I grabbed the moment and wrote a poem about nature—or was it about human nature?—about motion, time, and being alone, about how life changes around us, how we change in response, and the surprising possibilities for transformation.

MOTION AND TIME AND DRIVING ALONE

Everything changes in time.
I notice this approaching some barns
from the road—the road itself
moving under me.
A small red barn standing
to the left of a larger barn,
both in a green field, fields of corn,
some fenced in, but the green
and expanse of clouds,
the way the sun's light shadows the grasses,
my eyes fixed on that smaller barn,
the way it moves
from one side of the larger barn to the other.
The way it literally moved.
And my astonishment witnessing
what's impossible, like
the way I've changed.

POETRY PUBLICATIONS

Ebner's poetry publications include the following book:

The Space Between. Newton, Conn.: Hanover, 2000.

Ebner has poems published in the following journals:

Comstock Review; Fiddlesticks; IBIS; Register Citizen; Underwood Review.

Ebner's poetry is included in the following anthology:

Intensive Care: More Poetry and Prose by Nurses. Ed. Cortney Davis and Judy Schaefer. Iowa City: Univ. of Iowa Press, 2003.

Amy Haddad

ℰᴅ

Haddad weaves tales in her poems that create a tension between sophistication and simplicity. This tension is illustrated in her poem "Asking for Direction," which juxtaposes the complexities of medical care with the heretofore uncomplicated life of a woman whose husband had always made decisions for her. Nurses are the ones who are constantly in touch with the everyday realities of a patient's family. Having been a patient herself, Haddad understands how the demands of the medical profession often deflect doctors' and nurses' attention from the everyday reality of patients and their families. Haddad does what other patients do: she protects herself with talismans—and she suffers. She also does what poets do: she artfully uses language to give linguistic reference to the simple and sophisticated moments that are often nearly impossible to describe.

DEHISCENCE

You have come unstitched.
Holes appear on your threadbare abdomen.
Tunnels develop and connect bowel, liver, pancreas.
Enzymes ooze out and digest your skin,
no matter how hard we try to stem the flow.
Mounds of dressings,
miles of tape—a jerry-rigged system to
hold together our mistakes.
The stench is overwhelming, ever present
reminding everyone, but especially you,
that you have come undone.

Since I cannot bear your suffering,
since the truth is too horrible to grasp,
since I can offer you nothing else,

I clean you up.
I wash your face,
brush your teeth,
comb your hair,
turn you gently on your side,
push soiled linens away,
roll clean sheets under you,
remove layers and layers of damp, disgusting dressings,
and replace them with new dressings and tape.

Since I am helpless in the face of your tragedy,
I give you the certainty and calmness of my motions,
the competence and comfort of my touch

as I smooth the top sheet over my work.
Done.
For a few pristine moments, we allow ourselves
to be caught in the illusion of your wholeness.

In 1992 KATE BROWN, a colleague in the Center for Health Policy and Ethics at Creighton University, where I work, suggested we write a grant proposal to the state humanities council. The proposal was for a yearlong writing-group project involving women in health care. The project, "Logic of the Psyche: Health Care Ethics and Humanities," was funded by the Nebraska Humanities Council. The project was the catalyst for my creative writing about my life and work as a nurse. The group was not large, about ten, but diverse regarding our professions. Yet we all shared at least two things in common: we were all women and we wanted to explore a creative approach to the ethical issues we encountered in our clinical practice. We believed that literature could be a rich source of guidance to help identify and work through ethical dilemmas facing health professionals. We met every other week. Sometimes we met with facilitators who provided guidance in writing poetry, short stories, and drama. The rest of the time we met without a facilitator. The one constant for all our group meetings was that each member had to write something, not just talk about what we would like to write. We read parts of our work aloud, which was often a difficult thing to do. "Dehiscence" was one of my first pieces that grew out of the writing-group project.

The collective works of the writing group fell into three major themes in feminist perspectives in ethics: power and powerlessness, vulnerability and voice, and connection and disconnection. "Dehiscence" most clearly falls into the powerlessness category. The inspiration for the poem was the patients we could not fix—patients who were literally falling apart, despite our best efforts. I remembered patients like this who suffered horribly, not only in a physical sense but emotionally and psychologically too. The smell of decay and death hung heavy in their rooms.

The poem offers what little remedy there is to this tragedy: the presence of someone who isn't daunted by the sights and odors. Nurses seem to know when cure will not be achieved, yet see this not as a defeat but as a sign to move in closer. I never felt brave taking care of patients like this. I was often overwhelmed a   t, I found that even the m   ief respite not only for th   n "brief" respite, for no   e process repeats itself.

ASKING FOR DIRECTION

He fell dead in the parking lot of a convenient mart.

His wife never learned to drive,
had never written a check,
never made a move without asking him first.

And now they ask,
"What would you like us to do?"
"How aggressive should we be?"

And she tells them she must leave because
her neighbor is giving her a ride and it's her only way home.

When she visits again, they say,
"We suspect permanent brain damage.
Shall we resuscitate him if his heart stops beating?"

Day after day,
"Shall we discontinue the ventilator?"
"Shall we continue artificial nutrition and hydration?"
Waiting, she holds his limp hand,
silently begs him to tell her what to do.

Since he doesn't answer,
she slips out to catch a ride with her neighbor.

This poem was also born in the writing-group project. As an ethics consultant at several local hospitals, I listened to many cases like the one in the poem. I was struck by the number of family members, particularly women, who never made a serious decision in their lives without asking first for permission. Then, after a tragic accident or sudden illness of a loved one, they are asked to make life-and-death decisions for someone else. I wanted to convey the suddenness of death (thus the man dropping dead in a parking lot), the irony of this happening at a convenience store, and the heavy burden placed on a grieving, bewildered spouse.

I left the health professionals in the poem nameless and faceless, a sort of chorus. I wanted to convey the confusion that the wife was feeling and the urgency of the questions confronting her. Health-care professionals are programmed to ask these "routine" end-of-life questions that are anything but routine to patients and their families. The chorus repeatedly asks the wife questions she may not understand or just cannot answer. I purposefully left the technical jargon in to distance the wife from those who assume they are doing the right thing by honoring her wishes, her decision about what should happen to her husband.

The questions from the chorus increase in complexity, almost turning into a form of abandonment. Rather than helping her decide, the questions are posed and seem to hang there as the health professionals wait for an answer. I have heard physicians and nurses complain about family members like the wife, claiming that they are being resistant or in denial concerning the gravity of the situation. The wife's lack of transportation also takes on a negative connotation according to the staff. Is she trying to escape? Run away from her responsibilities? Or is this truly her only way to get home?

"Asking for Direction" has been used in many medical and nursing ethics courses as a sort of "counter story" to traditional end-of-life cases in ethics. It is particularly effective when one voice reads the narrator's part and a whole group reads the chorus, or when different voices read the questions one on top of the other. One immediately identifies with the wife, alone, grieving, and faced with an impossible decision. I almost want to slip out with her at the end of the poem.

GIRDING FOR BATTLE

The tiny, silver Celtic goddess
placidly hangs from a burgundy cord
around my neck.

She swings slightly
on a field of starched, white cotton.
My husband's shirt fastens the wrong way.
Awkwardly, I push the buttons
through the stiff holes.
A whiff of his scent lingers
Below the dry cleaner's efforts
as my body warms the fabric.
My last name stamped in black ink
inside his collar.
His scent.
My name.
His idea to wear the shirt—
easier to get on and off,
less painful to get my arm in the sleeve,
easier to wash off the blood and betadine.

So I wear these talismans
to protect me in the doctor's office.

While a member of the writing group, I was diagnosed with ductal carcinoma in situ and had to have a mastectomy and reconstructive surgery after numerous biopsies. Postoperatively, I had three drains in my chest and considerable swelling. None of my tops were loose enough, so my husband suggested I wear one of his slightly worn dress shirts. The shirt was big enough to cover everything and it wasn't as hard to get my affected arm in and out of the sleeve. My last name is different from my husband's. When I drop off his shirts at the cleaner, my name is stamped inside the collar. He has joked that this assures that he belongs to me.

I recently read an article asking various women to name their favorite piece of clothing. One young, petite woman chose her boyfriend's white T-shirt, stating, "He's so big that it comes down to my knees. It makes me feel safe." This sentiment is part of what I am trying to convey in the poem. When I got dressed to go to the doctor's office, especially right after surgery, I knew it would be painful and messy. Fluid collected under my skin around the surgical site, even with the drains in place, so the physician had to use a large syringe and a wide-bore needle to manually draw off this serosanginous fluid—hence the blood and betadine on my clothes.

I started to view these office visits with greater and greater dread. The image of arming or dressing for a battle seemed fitting to me as I prepared for yet one more trip to the surgeon's office. So I wore my husband's shirts and a silver necklace a friend gave me of the Celtic goddess for healing whenever I had to go to the doctor. My fear often caused me to heat up and get sweaty, which released my husband's scent—a combination of soap, aftershave, and his skin—that I saw as another source of protection. Also, I wanted to introduce a sensual image to connect my husband and me in stark contrast to the medical images. The "whiff" of sensuality and sexuality are just that, buried beneath the loss, pain, and dramatic changes to my body.

This is the first poem in which I played with the placement of words on the page. I wanted the reader to dwell on the word "linger" so the line breaks at that point. This poem also marks a shift in voice and perspective in my writing. It is written from a patient's view. I am now the one being acted upon, looking for ways to protect myself from the nameless, detached health professionals.

CHEMOTHERAPY LOUNGE

"I don't understand this. I only turned my back for a few seconds.
All our money was in there."

"Up next: Daydreaming about sex and why it's good for you."

The televisions talk for us,
fill the endless spaces.
There is no understanding.
Tacit treatment of cancer patients
who are all alike.
Lined up in lounge chairs,
at times almost fifty of us.

"Welcome back. We're talking about how to have house guests and enjoy them."

"What makes your adrenaline rush? What makes it pump?"

The faintly metallic odor of noxious drugs,
the sour-sweet overlay of vomit
permeates everything, even the carpet.
Trapped in our seats,
plugged to poles,
we sit for hours.
Poisoning takes time.

"It was to be a yearly lease but I let him have it month to month.
Then he wanted me to pay for the utilities.
I said, 'Do you want me to fix your breakfast, too?'"

"Let's get together tonight for dinner and finalize the details about the wedding."
"Sorry, Roxanne, not tonight."
"But darling, why?"

The nurse has on a felt pumpkin hat.
She sits heavily on a stool by my side,
drops ten or so filled syringes in her lap.
All of this will go into my body.
"So, how've you been?"
she asks without looking at me.
I feign sleep, try to shut out
noise and small talk.
Neither one of us is really here.
Magenta adriamycin crawls
up the tubing to the port
just above my bra.

"Tanya, welcome to our show. Tell us why things haven't been going so well between
you and Roger."

"Storms will fire up here—expect some wind damage;
it'll juice up down south with heavy rain."

The taste of the drug
hits me as soon
as it slips past the port.
My tongue itches.
I whisper,
"I'm so sick."
A reflex pat on the arm,
emesis basin and towel in reply.

"Now your clothes can smell like you just hung them out to dry in the sunshine."

"When are you going to tell him the baby isn't his?"

What I need
is a large-breasted woman—
pale, yellow house dress
worn, blue plaid apron.
I catch the scent of Vel soap
as she enfolds me on her old porch glider.
Bridal wreath in full bloom
shades us as we rock back and forth.

She rubs my back
with a depth of compassion I can collapse in
and never bottom out
while she softly repeats,
"What a terrible thing to happen to you, honey.
What a terrible thing."

Six years after my first mastectomy, I was diagnosed with invasive carcinoma, stage IIA. This time I not only had a mastectomy, but I also had to undergo six months of chemotherapy. I received chemotherapy every three weeks in a large outpatient clinic. When I wasn't getting treatment, I still had to be there every week for lab work. I grew to hate walking in the door of the clinic. The smells, the waiting room full of sick and fearful patients and their families were almost more than I could bear. All the patients receiving chemotherapy sat in groups of four, facing each other with a television for each group. Each TV would invariably be on a different station (thanks to cable, many different stations) and turned up to drown out the noise from the next group's TV. I wanted to capture the cacophony of voices and the contrast between the banalities on TV with what was happening in the "lounge."

Like most patients, I had an indwelling venous access device placed in my chest, just above my bra on the left side. I still don't know why, but this made me feel so vulnerable. After the first treatment, I was only mildly sick. Of course I lost my hair during this time, so it was a blessing not to have to deal with nausea too. The overwhelming nausea came after the second treatment. I had heard of patients who got sick just thinking of going in for chemotherapy and never understood this. Now I did.

The matter-of-fact attitude of the nurses upset and disappointed me. All of them were kind; that wasn't the problem. It was the fact that this was routine for them, not for me. Even though I knew why I was getting the drugs, how they worked, and what was supposed to happen, knowledge wasn't enough to get me through this. The lack of privacy for something I considered private was almost as bad as the treatment. If a patient vomited, there were no curtains to draw, so everyone in your group shared in the event. And just like grade school, when one person got sick, others soon followed. During my third treatment, I vomited all over my clothes. I got sick so fast there was no warning. The nurses gave me scrubs to change into and put my soiled clothes in a plastic bag. This was the nadir for me.

I wanted to convey how crowded and open to scrutiny the patients were but contrast it with the "spaces" between us (patients and nurses) in terms of emotional distance and understanding. I wrote to remember the sights, sounds, and smells and what this felt like.

The last two stanzas grew out of a conversation with a friend to whom I was complaining about treatment and how it was delivered. She asked, "What do you want the nurses to do, Amy?" I thought about this a lot and still do. Maybe my expectation was too great or misplaced. What I wanted was a place to pour out my pain, a place to lean, and a shoulder to sigh and sob into. At the least, I wanted the recognition that this wasn't just another day at work for me, that something of significance was happening here.

I began to write poetry around the age of nine or ten. I recently found one of my first poems about the Easter bunny and was amused at the rhymes I must have struggled to create. The next poem I remember writing was a haiku: "Gentle butterfly, fragile bit of summer air, melting into sky." We learned about the structure of Japanese poetry in eighth grade and this was my attempt at the form. I remember being encouraged to write poetry and fiction all through my grade-school and high-school days. I have always found poetry to be the truest expression of my feelings, fears, hopes, and secrets.

I read almost anything as a child. The first books I remember reading on my own were by Dr. Seuss. I liked the rhythm and words. *Alice in Wonderland* and *Through the Looking Glass* by Lewis Carroll remain favorites. I enjoyed the drama, romance, and unusual language of the Brontë sisters in *Jane Eyre* and *Wuthering Heights*. Poets who have influenced my work are twentieth-century American poets e.e. cummings and Anne Sexton, and contemporary American poet Tess Gallagher.

My mother loves poetry and committed many poems to memory from a book my grandmother gave her when she was in high school. At an early age, I'd listen to bits and pieces of poems that she would recite as she cleaned or washed dishes. The one I liked the best was called "Dried Apple Pies" (author long ago forgotten), and I can still recall the first line of the poem: "I loathe, abhor, detest, despise, abominate dried apple pies." I loved the rhythm of the words, building the emotion with the number of syllables. The rhythm caught my attention before I really understood the words. I was fascinated by the way the author made the reader pause for a beat after the word "abominate," as if to keep the reader waiting just a little more before learning the focus of this hatred, even though the poet never used the word "hate." Finally, I loved the juxtaposition of these strong emotions with such a mundane object. It is my first and favorite for all of these reasons, yet I hold other poems almost as dear for different reasons; among these are "i thank You God for most this amazing / day," by e.e. cummings and "Let Evening Come" by recently deceased contemporary American poet Jane Kenyon.

What keeps me writing? I think this question is really "what keeps me *from* writing?" Somehow there is always something else calling for my attention and time that takes me away from writing. I know that it is the only work that truly comes from me and everything and everyone who made me who I am. Since my work in ethics education doesn't require creative writing, I continue to try to find time on the side to remain a poet.

POETRY PUBLICATIONS

Haddad's poetry publications include the following book:

The Arduous Touch: Women's Voices in Health Care. Co-editor. West Lafayette, Ind.: Purdue Univ. Press, 1999. An anthology of stories and poems by women health-care professionals.

Haddad has poems published in the following journals:

American Journal of Nursing; Fetishes; Journal of General Internal Medicine; Journal of Medical Humanities; Reflections on Professional Nursing.

Haddad's poetry is included in the following anthologies:

The Arduous Touch: Women's Voices in Health Care. Ed. Amy Haddad and Kate Brown. West Lafayette, Ind.: Purdue Univ. Press, 1999.
Between the Heartbeats: Poetry and Prose by Nurses. Ed. Cortney Davis and Judy Schaefer. Iowa City: Univ. of Iowa Press, 1995.
Intensive Care: More Poetry and Prose by Nurses. Ed. Cortney Davis and Judy Schaefer. Iowa City: Univ. of Iowa Press, 2003.

Veneta Masson

ℰ

Masson's poetry creates islands of time. The reader will feel on the move with Masson, an elegant poet who knows how to travel. Whether describing a safe house, how to be at home, or a personal journey with her sister, these poems take us places we have never been before and bring us back home with images and memories to savor. Masson's imaginative life begins with and is sustained by the gift of her grandmother's continuing presence in her life. Although no one can truly teach us how to live and die, Masson comes close—if we read carefully. Furthermore Masson teaches us how to prepare, and how to pack.

WHAT'S THERE IN GRANDMA'S DIARY

What's there is mostly
what she bought, how much she paid
every home perm she got or gave
long distance phone calls
trips out of town
big events like the end of the war
boys coming home, births, deaths
the election of Presidents.

I am there, too—
how, at one, I made noise like a fish
how, at four, I learned to say L's
and how, at six, I came up with
cute names for the baby.

Combing for clues, I've pinned
some memories down to real time—

the Cleveland tornado
John's terrible nosebleed—
and got to the root of a few
familiar tangles. Still,
so much has been suppressed.

Aside from blind maternal pride
any inkling of how she felt
is blotted out indelibly.
I hold the frayed pages up
to the light to try to see
what's beneath. Exclamation points
poke through here and there
but nothing of what provoked them.

I think how very like her I am,
first committing my life to words
then reneging. Why?
a change of heart,
prudent regard
or a primitive fear
of what's been unleashed to prowl
and run amok between the lines?

"GRANDMA'S DIARY" IS ONE of a score of poems I wrote during the months I was reeling from the impact of a guided imagery session in which I discovered just how much my maternal grandmother meant to me. I spent the first years of my life in her home while my father was stationed in England during World War II. My mother used to tell me my birth story each year: that cold Sunday night in February when she and Grandma listened to Phil Spitalny and his All-Girl Orchestra on the radio, the snowy taxi ride to the hospital, the long, ethery labor and delivery, my status in the nursery—the only girl, the nurses' "rose among thorns," and those first anxious days and nights in my grandmother's house with both women keeping watch over my cradle.

Even after my mother and father were reunited and we moved to Cleveland from a small town on Lake Erie, Grandma and I continued to have a special relationship. She'd spend time in our home and I in hers. Between visits, we'd correspond. In letters, I was always her friend of so many years, months, and days, dating from the day I was born. "So how's my friend of ten years, two months, and five days?" was her standard greeting. I'd check her math, make sure she was right. In her last letter to me, her friend of twenty-four years, three months, and seven days, she sends the latest news, advises me on packing for my much-anticipated "maiden voyage" to Europe ("Jersey . . . would make a nice traveling dress") and tells me about her plans to return to Ohio from my parents' home in California. As always, she signed her letter "Herran haltuun [Finnish for 'in the hands of the Lord'], With love, Gram, 'Bye."

Just weeks into my trip, she had a stroke, then another, after which she died. "There's nothing you can do," my mother said, trying to console me long distance from California to the train station in Luxembourg. I cried, wanting to go home, to go—somehow—to my grandmother. But there was my traveling companion to think of, and the two years we'd spent saving for this journey. I decided to continue on. By the time I returned to the States months later, the family had worked through its grief. I had merely buried mine.

What a surprise I had in store, twenty-odd years later, when I opened the lid of the imaginary treasure chest I dug up with the imaginary shovel propped against a tall tree deep in my imaginary woods and found—stacks of paper. Stacks of paper! Were they poems, perhaps, or deeds or banknotes? The therapist who was guiding me saw my mind at work and reminded me, "Don't make it up; just see what you see." So I cleared my mental screen and waited for an image to appear.

> *Imagine!*
> *They are letters!*
> *Letters from your grandmother*
> *bundled and tied*
> *before she died*
> *against the time*
> *you'd find them.*
>
> *Imagine*
> *Grandma*
> *speaking to you*
> *from the deepest place*
> *where imagination*
> *and memory*
> *have their common source*
> *in the springbed of truth.*

I stumbled home from this session, overwhelmed with grief, realizing that I'd never said goodbye to this person who taught me the meaning of love and adventure. I pored over her photos, letters, and the paintings that hung in my house. (In her sixties, she took up oil painting; I used to accompany her to her art class.) My favorite of these showed, from the rear, a horse-drawn sleigh stopping by woods on a snowy evening. You see the figures of an adult and child. A grandfather—no, a grand*mother*—and grandchild. Here we were, enshrined as characters in a Robert Frost poem.

I don't recall just when the first of what I call my grandmother poems came, but working with them occupied me steadily for months to the exclusion of all other creative work. I'm like this. I focus on one theme, one project at a time. As in guided imagery, you don't know where you're headed when you begin to write a poem. You clear your mental screen and wait for an image to appear. But even in the later stages, as you wrestle with form and word choices, there are revelations. During this period, my mother sent me Grandma's diary. I'd never seen it before. A little larger than an index card and less than an inch thick, only half of its brown leather cover and binding remained. It was held together by a brown rubber band, just like the ones my grandmother always kept handy around her wrist. The brief jottings in this tattered "Five-Year Diary" spanned several decades. When I started ruminating about my grandmother's entries and what they might tell me about her, I hadn't a clue that I would also gain some insights into myself (*how very like her I am*). In this poem, for example, even as I speculate about passages she had blotted out and her reasons for reneging on what she had written, I got in touch with my own ambivalence about "committing my life to words" and my "primitive fear / of what's been unleashed / to prowl and run amok / between the lines."

I possessed a locked diary for a brief spell when I was a young teen, but can't remember trusting any facts or feelings of personal importance to its pages. Even now, I take refuge in the concision, innuendo, and layers of meaning that a good poem allows—demands. In a poem, I reveal and conceal at the same time. When readers tell me, "I've had that same experience" or "I felt just like you did," I'm reminded that the universal lies embedded in the particular.

I have a vivid memory of myself at age six, sitting on my bed and writing a poem inspired by a plaque on the bedroom wall that read, "Put God First." That one poem, soon lost, constituted my entire output in childhood. Inspired by love, boredom, or melancholy, I wrote a few poems in my twenties, but it was in my thirties that I started to write regularly and undertook learning the craft.

The only stories that I remember being read to me as a child were Bible stories. Perhaps that's why biblical imagery often finds its way into my writing. Once I learned to read, my favorite poets seem to have been Mother Goose and, the one that intrigued me most, Anonymous. I have collected—and discarded—many other favorites along the way. Those that will always sustain and delight me include Langston Hughes, Chilean poet Gabriela Mistral, Derek Walcott, Mary Oliver, Linda Pastan, and my friend and frequent first reader Cheryl Hellner.

Reading and writing are two important ways I've come to understand myself and the larger world. I like to think of my writing as soul food that I hope will bring nourishment, comfort, and pleasure to the reader, just as other poets have created a feast for me. In my thirties, I started to keep a written journal. It has been the seedbed for many of my poems and essays. I still keep one, though only when the spirit moves. I find that I use fewer words (snippets rather than narratives) and more visual expressions—mandalas, sketches, symbols, collages, and images from dreams and what I call my soulscape, the parallel world I inhabit in my imagination. I write regularly and with discipline but have no routine. I have to wait for an energy surge. This usually occurs in the morning during periods when I have a sufficient amount of what playwright August Wilson called *brain space*. Like other writers, I'm always composing something in my head, but most of it ends up in that rich compost heap of the imagination.

THE SECRET LIFE OF NURSES

You won't read about it in the tabloids
or inside the gaudy jacket of a Harlequin.
Dear Abby knows nothing about it.
Priests and lovers may think they do
and you
as you glimpse the tips of their shoes
        stalled outside a door—
you may think you do,
but you don't.

Nurses keep a safe house hidden
in the spaciousness of imagination—
    a dark kiva dug into
            the sun-bleached cliff
    a gracious ark
            gliding high on still waters
    a lavender planet idling among far stars.

They keep a safe house
and a fleet of neurons poised for flight.

When my friend Doris told me, "I don't like poetry, but I like your poems," I took it as a great compliment. Although I want my poems to be well crafted and memorable, I also want them to be accessible and meaningful to the casual reader. I want them to work for a living and make their own way in the world. So when Doris read "The Secret Life of Nurses" and said with characteristic candor, "I don't understand any of it," I was disappointed. Doris was a nurse, after all. Didn't she have some sort of safe house like I do? Where did *she* go when the cares and stresses of nursing caught up with her?

Ten years ago, I wrote an essay for the *American Journal of Nursing* titled "My Life as a Symptom" in which I described some of my trials as nurse and director of a small, inner-city clinic in Washington, D.C. In it, I divulged the fact that I kept a fantasy apartment in Cairo overlooking the Nile where I daydreamed, wrote, and entertained a select circle of artists and cosmopolites. I'd jet there after work or on weekends after a rough week. I loved that place, deciding that it represented the life I was really meant to live. Although this particular place existed only in my imagination, I'd once been entertained in one very like it back in the days when I was traveling to exotic places as director of nursing for an international health organization.

That life may as well have been a fantasy, too, compared to the grit and mire in which I became enmeshed as a hands-on nurse. *Real life* in our clinic consisted of a web of patients and families with insoluble problems, coworkers as committed as I but with whom I didn't always see eye to eye, a bank account running on empty, health-care financing and referral systems broken beyond repair, middle-of-the-night phone calls, middle-of-the-day nightmares, and nowhere to hide. Or was there? Ah, Cairo!

Perhaps the poem started with the image of a nurse stalled outside a door. In retrospect I see that I've used that image at least once before, in a poem titled "Passages." In it, I wrote about being in charge of the care of a forty-year-old woman, dying of uterine cancer, whose "difficult" husband was a gynecologist on the staff of the hospital where I worked.

> *At 20, I was a novice still*
> > *and ill at ease*
> > *with the celebration*
> > *of mysteries.*
> *Reluctantly, I began my rounds, knowing that door*
> > *at the end of the hall*
> > *was one I had to open.*

Sometimes, as in the poe[...] through but most
of us professional caregi[...]
of Ben and Jerry's New [...]
the gym, or a trip to "a l[...]
respite and renewal. Ho[...]
of neurons poised for flight."

METASTASIS

from Late Latin, transition,
from Greek, meta- (involving change) + histanai (cause to stand)

The trip to Paradise
was planned well before
the recurrence
manifested itself
cunningly
like sleight of hand—
now here, now there—
among the once vital
organs.

After a brief flurry of indecision—
more-chemo-what-the-hell
or a peek at Paradise—
she chose the latter
as having perhaps the better claim
because it was classy
and wouldn't she fare
a lot better on an island in the sun
than head down in a toilet bowl
flushed
with toxins?

Knowing how way leads on to way
she went
and, sure enough,
basking there
in Paradise,
she sighed and said
If only I never had to go back . . .

I tell you this: metastasis
was a magical word
before cancer
got hold of it.
It could transform you.
Still can.

THE SILENCE OF DOLLHOOD

She: Homecoming Princess Forever
I: Savvy Globetrotting Grad

See how we tried to shrinkwrap each other
like costumed Barbies
kept on a shelf for display.

And now we sit
in a shelter by the sea
over late morning coffee

She: Ill Princess
I: Failed Grad

both of us fallen from safety,
stripped of our cellophane wrappers.

How, in this small island of time,
to redeem the silence of dollhood
take up our voices
and storm the family plot?

Let death not be
the only denouement.

During the years my sister was living with cancer, just after the official diagno-
sis of recurrent metastatic breast cancer had been conferred, a book found its
way to me. It was titled *Remarkable Recovery—What Extraordinary Healings
Tell Us about Getting Well and Staying Well*, by Caryle Hirshberg and Marc

Ian Barasch. In it, the authors set out to investigate the phenomenon of unex-
plained remission from cancer with the same rigor as scientists who study its
pathology and treatment. Surely, they suggested, there is as much or more to be
learned from long-term, disease-free survivors as from those in the throes of
illness. I devoured the book and quickly sent a copy to my sister. Although the
authors never offered a recipe for recovery, I latched onto the book—the title
page would have been enough—as a sort of talisman. Spontaneous remission
does occur. Let Rebecca be blessed with a remarkable recovery.

She was not. Like most women in her situation, she died. As I continue to
ponder my own experience of her illness, I sometimes think I ought to write
a book titled *Remarkable Recurrences.* For example, the tacit knowledge that
we sisters were saying hello to good-bye resulted in our taking a series of trips
together, trips we would never have thought possible otherwise, in which we
were able to break what I have come to think of as the "silence of dollhood."
"See how we tried to shrinkwrap each other / like costumed Barbies / kept
on a shelf for display," I wrote in one of many poems that helped me wrest
meaning from the events of those years. I'd always played the role of savvy,
globe-trotting older sister. She'd been the homecoming princess who married
the prince, settled down, had kids, and lived happily ever after. We hardly knew
each other. It took a life-threatening illness to propel us toward intimacy.

By the time we traveled to Paradise Island in the Bahamas, Rebecca was
beginning to have severe headaches. An ominous sign. Should she do another
course of chemotherapy? Perhaps, but certainly not before she'd seen Paradise!
Besides the trip itself, there were two other seeds that gave rise to the poem
"Metastasis." One was the original meaning of the word. Like the poet I am,
I went first to the dictionary rather than to the scientific literature for under-
standing. I was not disappointed. This "terrible" word actually derives from
Latin and Greek for transition, change, to cause to stand. How wonderful!

The second seed was Robert Frost's poem "The Road Not Taken" in which
the poet uses the metaphor of a fork in the road to describe how the simplest
of choices can have a profound effect on our future.

> *Two roads diverged in a wood, and I—*
> *I took the one less traveled by,*
> *and that has made all the difference.*

Some of the lines in "Metastasis" are riffs on Frost's, a tribute to his genius and
evidence of how his poetic imagination sparked mine.

LA MUERTE

If Muerte comes and sits down beside you,
you are lucky, because Death has chosen
to teach you something.
—CLARISSA PINKOLA ESTES

Old Mother Death sits
down beside me.
Neither cruel nor kind
she does not take, she receives.
We are, all of us, her wards.
Contrary to what you may think
she is in no hurry.
Only humans fret about time.
She squats close to the earth
knees spread wide in a generous lap
and there, mossy shawl drawn
close about her, she waits, shuffling
the letters of her strange alphabet.
I see her fingerpads smudged with ink.
I edge closer.
I am ready to learn.

I've been a nurse for over thirty-five years—in hospitals, homes, hospices. I've closed eyelids in death. I've shared the grief of many families, including my ny patients who, at the end en Rebecca was diagnosed ly toward a deeper intimacy and mine—and that it had

Poetry was the strong medicine I used to cope with fear, anger, and despair. I searched out poems that expressed the feelings I couldn't and, on days I was unable to pray or pick up the phone, I'd send her one of them. Let these poets earn their keep, I reasoned. Let them speak for me. Because it is my way, I also began to write poems out of my experience of my sister's illness. The first of these dates from the evening before her mastectomy. I'd just arrived for a visit, completely unprepared for news of the breast lump (discovered in the course of a routine annual exam) and ominous pathology report. Now Rebecca and I sat on her bedroom floor, doors closed against the sounds of children and an as-yet-undisrupted household—two sisters alone together, saying hello to goodbye.

After her death, I was flooded with images—of her, of us, of the times we'd spent together in pursuit of treatment or respite during the three-and-a-half-year course of her illness, and of the events that marked her final days. One afternoon during that first year of grieving, I remember listening to an audio-tape by Clarissa Pinkola Estes (*The Creative Fire*) in which she said, "If Muerte comes and sits down beside you, you are lucky, because Death has chosen to teach you something" (Boulder, Colo., *Sounds True* audiotape). Indeed.

I decided I wanted to meet this Muerte. So one day I simply sat in my room, took a few deep breaths, closed my eyes, entered my imagination, and waited for Muerte to appear. My first surprise, as the image came into focus on my mental screen, was that Death was no dark, rapacious male, slyly snatching our loved ones away. No. She—*she!*—was an old grandmother—*Grandmother!*—sitting in the thick woods at the edge of perception, patiently waiting for *us* to come to *her*. I stayed with the imagery as long as I could, absorbing details and sensations. The experience not only enlarged my understanding, it changed the quality of my grief for my sister. It was a great gift. Grandma speaking to me—"from the deepest place."

That a poem would come was inevitable. I needed some vessel to contain this new knowledge—something more suitable than a hastily scribbled journal entry describing an experience in a realm beyond language. As always, the poet's craft, which guided my choices of words, sounds, and structure, enhanced rather than distorted the original imagery. In "La Muerte," Old Mother Death is there as I saw her. *I edge closer. I am ready to learn.*

POETRY PUBLICATIONS

Masson's poetry publications include the following books:

Rehab at the Florida Avenue Grill. Washington, D.C.: Sage Femme, 1999.
Just Who. Washington, D.C.: Crossroad Health Ministry, 1993.

Masson has poems published in the following journals:

American Journal of Nursing; Annals of Internal Medicine; International Journal of Human Caring; Journal of Medical Humanities; Journal of the American Medical Association; Mediphors; Natural Bridge; Nursing and Health Care Perspectives; Nursing Spectrum; Potomac Review; The Sun.

Masson's poetry is included in the following anthologies:

The Arduous Touch: Women's Voices in Health Care. Ed. Amy Haddad and Kate Brown. W. Lafayette, Ind.: NotaBell, 1999.

Between the Heartbeats: Poetry and Prose by Nurses. Ed. Cortney Davis and Judy Schaefer. Iowa City: Univ. of Iowa Press, 1995.

The Cancer Poetry Project: Poems by Cancer Patients and Those Who Love Them. Ed. Karin B. Miller. Minneapolis: Fairview, 2001.

Community Health Nursing: Caring for Populations. 4th ed. Mary Jo Clark. Upper Saddle River, N.J.: Prentice Hall, 2002.

The HeART of Nursing: Expressions of Creative Art in Nursing. Ed. Cecilia Wendler. Indianapolis: Center for Nursing, 2002.

Hungry as We Are: An Anthology of Washington Area Poets. Ed. Ann Darr. Washington, D.C.: Washington Writers, 1995.

Intensive Care: More Poetry and Prose by Nurses. Ed. Cortney Davis and Judy Schaefer. Iowa City: Univ. of Iowa Press, 2003.

A Life in Medicine: A Literary Anthology. Ed Robert Coles and Randy Testa. New York: New Press, 2002.

Nursing in the Community: Dimensions of Community Health Nursing. Mary Jo Clark. 2d and 3d eds. Stamford, Conn.: Appleton and Lange, 1996, 1999.

On Being a Doctor. Ed. Michael A. LaCombe. Philadelphia: American College of Physicians, 1995.

100 Years of American Nursing. Ed. Thelma M. Schorr and Mary Shaun Kennedy. Philadelphia: Lippincott, 1999.

Unbearable Uncertainty. Ed. Amy Bowes, Terry S. Gingras, Beth A. Kaplowitt, and Anne Perkins. Northampton, Mass.: Pioneer Valley Breast Cancer Network, 2000.

Uncharted Lines: Poems from the Journal of the American Medical Association. Ed. Charlene Breedlove. Albany, Calif.: Boaz, 1998.

Lianne Elizabeth Mercer

৪৯

Mercer, a certified poetry therapist, writes to record and remember, "to keep,"
she says, "what [her] heart has learned." One has the sense that Mercer can
barely stop writing poetry long enough to tell us about her poems and poetry
therapy. She practices what she teaches others about the healing power of poetry.
Mercer shares the death of her mother in intimate detail and takes us along on
her cathartic journey into Canyon de Chelly in the poem "Sunrise." In this par-
ticular poem, the canyon becomes organic, alive, and changing, with red walls
and the "slow smile" of the morning sun. There is a geographical sense of place
in her poems—and a metaphorical sense of place as well. In colorful and precise
language, Mercer reminds us that the biggest surprises are usually in our own
proverbial backyards.

BENEDICIÓN

In Room 28, an old woman perches on her bed
stiff with fear. She licks crooked, gold-filled teeth,
spews Spanish words of sorrow that fall like tears.
I hold out my hands like sieves dripping syllables, say
No comprendo. Ah, she makes the sign of the cross.
Her long fingers reach for mine.

She smiles around my tentative use of *dolor* and *las flores,*
words spoken on this dusky evening eventual night will extinguish.
She enriches me—reveals me to myself growing in a dawn garden
where zinnias reach for the sun with mariachi arms, where
clicking beetles make music far sweeter than excuses of language
blooming, then fading, in our hands.

I breathe in this gift of recognition
from a bent-over woman whose heart bursts
with words needing no voice, spilling
from her eyes into mine, dancing now
beneath our fingers, affirming that we are kin,
breath of feathers on my arm, whispers in my soul.

THE MEMORY OF THE ELDERLY HISPANIC WOMAN'S shining eyes and her touch stayed with me for weeks. So did her smile. I wrote this poem to remember the special feelings I had when I thought about her. And to remind me of the connections we all want to make with our patients—connections of caring, respect, and service.

Writing this poem was an affirmation of something I have long believed and seen: we are all connected, whether or not we share the same language. We can let lack of a common language divide us and keep us apart, or we can find interpreters or take instruction in the language. When there isn't "touching" with words, we can go beyond language to physical touch, to the sparkle in the eye, to the smile, and to the mysterious and very real connection we have to each other as human beings.

I believe in keeping the mystery.

Writing poetry also demands that I keep that mystery. Writing, I enter into an intuitive relationship with what wants to be said. I hope for that time when language will lead me into a surprising meaning I hadn't realized before, a child of a meaning dancing just out of sight, affirming my humanity and telling me I'm in synch with the universe. I can explain poetic devices—simile, metaphor, alliteration, and paradox. I can tell a sonnet from a ghazal and have written both. I know the beat of iambic pentameter. But when I write, I put that momentarily aside and let the words invade my bones and reside in my heart. I quiet my mind and listen for the poem that's trying to find me. When words first spill onto the page, I see the shape the poem wants to take. One word per line. Rhyme. Long lines. Short ones. Stanzas.

Craft and my need for closure disappear, and I am alone with the exhilarating, mysterious gifts that language brings. I liken it to interacting with my patients. I explain procedures to them. I teach them about health and medications. Then, in a leap of faith, I feel an unspoken invitation to transcend what I scientifically "know," and I act on what I believe in my heart, what I feel in my body to be true. By some miracle, some chemistry, my heart connects to a place in the patient's heart that invites healing.

I find it fascinating that with so much of my energy devoted to language, "Bendición" sought me when there was an absence of language that might have delivered a gift of healing. I believe if I am listening, the poem will come.

Sometimes it delivers words. Sometimes healing takes another path.

When I say "healing," I don't necessarily mean that an illness will be cured. I mean a healing of the spirit, one soul touching another soul, affirming what connections the gift of life has provided for each of us. I mean being willing to be vulnerable, to say what we notice or feel and not expect certain answers. I mean creating a space between me and another person where our hearts and minds can leap into unexpected, rewarding, heart-wrenching places where we are moved, sometimes to tears and despair and other times to joy and laughter.

To me, healing is about relinquishing control and inviting in the unexpected, the mysterious. It happens when a patient realizes things he or she didn't understand before. It happens when I realize things I didn't understand before. The potential of that spark between the patient and me is when I feel most like a nurse, relating to a patient on a deeper level. Nurse and patient, we teach each other.

The progression of "Benedición" is about affirming our common humanity. Through our exchange and through the writing of this poem, I saw that it was an accident of circumstance that this woman was the patient and I was the nurse. I saw, through her eyes, that what she wanted is what I also want for myself—to be understood.

To touch and be touched. Touching is a primitive way of communicating that has no universal meaning and can often be misinterpreted. So much depends on body language and intent. Touching can be a simple acknowledgment of another's presence, an act of aggression, an arousal of sexual desire, or a desire for comfort and physical closeness. Our mothers touched us as infants; often, in adulthood, depending on our cultural values, we touch less. We say "We've lost touch" or "We're out of touch." Yet touching is what we want when we're sick or in danger. And it's what we want to give when we sense another's despair.

When my mother was in the nursing home, one of the pleasures of her day was when I rubbed lotion on her face, held her hand to file her nails, bathed her, or rubbed her back. She was not a "toucher" or a "hugger," but she loved being touched in these simple ways. It was something I could do for her when there was little left that I could do. We do not know who will teach us best, or in what circumstances. I took a long look at my own willingness to touch and be touched. I understand the professional prohibitions. Yet this moment of touching and being touched was a healing one.

The profession of nursing is not what it was when Florence Nightingale fought rats and ignorance in the Crimea nearly 150 years ago and returned to England to help shatter many established modes of treatment. For increased knowledge about better health and better ways of accomplishing that, I am grateful.

Classmates at the University of Michigan School of Nursing wrote a song called "Flo Never Had It So Good." We sang it on our journey through nursing school. We continue to sing it at reunions. What do we have that's better than what Flo had? Acknowledgment that we are a profession with skills and machines Flo never dreamed of. But we have the same obligation to care for patients that she had. She called it an art. More often than I would like, it seems to me that we don't have time to integrate the art, the science, the mystery, and the surprises of healing as our patients live out their illnesses. This inattention to meaning, this hurry-up syndrome makes us cranky. It interferes not only with our ability to care for patients but with caring for ourselves and each other.

The benediction of the Hispanic woman's touch reminds me how important touching is. In the last stanza of the poem, I wanted to talk about how the gift of touch is given and received. It occurred to me to begin with breath. There are so many expressions related to the breath—we catch our breath in awe, we hold our breath in anger, we breathe in a pleasing odor, and the space between our first and last breath is one of the boundaries of our lives. I liked the feelings evoked by the words, "I breathe in this gift of recognition." I wanted to circle back to the first stanza's images of hands with different images. I laughed when I was handed the gift of the last words, the softness of the "breath of feathers on my arm, whispers in my soul." Breath. Whispers. Elusive. Lovely, paradoxical metaphors for the unbreakable human bond.

Laughter and creativity touch. The writing process holds out its hands to be touched by trust. The result is "Benedición." This poem has given me a picture of my mind in a moment of attention to something important, and I am grateful.

EXILES

They come wearing relief
and apology, dressed in ragged jeans
or wrinkled khakis. They come
wearing bewilderment and anger
dressed in black T-shirts
and faded dreams.

These young men are suspicious,
now, of everyone, including
themselves. They've tried booze
and marijuana, sex and sleep.
Nothing—not even mother,

especially not mother—can sew up
the fraying edges of their thoughts.

Something has invaded their minds.
Birds have begun to nest on ideas
in trees bare of intention. Thoughts
branch into tangled whispers,
shouts for fertilizer or bug spray.
Words change meanings, demeaning,
demanding attention.

From lives of failed perspective,
the stories fall. The young men
look inward and outward at the same time,
walk the narrow bridge medication provides
between worlds. They remind us
we cannot go home again.
We must always walk head on
into the foreign countries of our lives.

I wrote this poem the same night I admitted two young men in their twenties to a psychiatric intensive care unit. One young man had been diagnosed as bipolar a couple years before. He'd been in the hospital twice since that time, had taken/abandoned medication, and had relapsed. The other, a college student, had been told by his physician that he was schizophrenic, which sent him into a profound depression. In their faces and in the faces of their parents, I saw such sorrow, bewilderment, and anger that I had to find a container for it. I found this poem.

Or rather, as I fervently believe, this poem found me. It provided a place to put anguish on the page—theirs and mine. To not forget and to honor these patients' lives in a profound way that will live for me past their discharge. To find joy. Sometimes buried so deeply that it seems not to be there, like an iris bulb under the snow. Sometimes playing tricks on the mind, like fireflies flitting in a confusing dance. Sometimes whistling an elusive tune in the dark of depression and despair, opposite feelings and images that invite the senses.

That night I found myself wearing the mantle of sorrow, of recognition that life doesn't give us what we expect, though it hands us ways to cope so we don't go under. I wondered how I would handle a similar situation if it were to occur in my family. I believed that giving words to this agony, this disappointment, this disrupted chaotic time in these young men's lives, in their family's lives, would lead me to greater compassion and understanding. It did. I was disappointed that, though I wrote the poem before morning, I didn't have the opportunity to share it with either of these young men or their families.

One of the beauties of poetry is that it invites paradox, the stuff our lives are made of. In *Poetic Medicine, The Healing Art of Poem-Making* (New York: Jeremy P. Tarcher/Putnam, 1997, p. 12) author John Fox quotes Peggy Osna Heller, a registered poetry therapist: "Poetic language honors polarities. We use the language of poetry to provide the many levels of feeling, facets of knowing, simultaneously, so we can examine them and move forward." We do not live totally in depression or anger, though it sometimes seems that way. Writing a poem lets me find hope in unexpected places—lets me find a larger meaning than that which exists in the situation itself.

I was open to whatever language the process of writing the poem would provide. Bewilderment, anger, and "faded dreams" came in words with hard "g," "d," and "b" sounds. In the last stanza, words with "w" came, which is a softer sound. I felt my feelings shift from frustration and despair to the possibility of hope for these young men's futures. I wanted to tell them this, but everyone was sleepy. Parents left with relief. The young men fell into bed and into the arms of Morpheus with the help of Ambien and Dalmane. I realized that while I was writing this poem before the end of the shift, I had seen a larger picture. That picture includes increasing hope for myself when I acknowledge my own bravery by exploring the foreign country of my life.

When "Exiles" was published in the *American Journal of Nursing*, caregivers and parents of similarly afflicted young men wrote to tell me that I'd put their feelings into words. Part of the joy of writing poetry is sensing thoughts and feelings others feel but can't articulate and putting them on the page. Most of the time weeks pass before I write the poem, so I don't share these poems with those I'm writing about. I wish I could. Perhaps as part of the discharge paperwork, we could give patients a poem that would be equally as important as a prescription—heart and mind medicine, acknowledgment that patients and their families have been heard.

The devices of poetry that I found most useful in writing this poem, besides paradox, were metaphor and the language itself, which handed me words I wouldn't have thought of, had not a phrase, a notion, a gesture triggered them.

"They come wearing relief / and apology," combined with the description of their actual clothes, allowed the images to expand, to become more than the words indicated. "Birds have begun to nest on ideas / in trees bare of intention" refers to their sad feelings of alienation. At the end of the third stanza, I wanted to write words that confuse and frighten—flights of ideas and sounds morphing into themselves without apparent meaning. Yet meaning is always there.

I once admitted a sixty-year-old man who had been schizophrenic for more than thirty years and had been in and out of the state hospital and other hospitals. He had few teeth and looked disheveled. He was here now because his thirty-eight-year-old retarded daughter had died the week before. He and his wife had cared for her. He was so despondent over her death that he wanted to kill himself. No one's life is ordinary. The details and the dignity astound and nourish me.

I write to remember lives that have touched mine in ways they could not have imagined. In the rush of admissions at 3:00 A.M., I don't expect to be inspired with a poem. I do expect, however, to keep open the possibility of seeing with the heart what is invisible to the eye, as the fox told the little prince in Antoine de Saint-Exupéry's *The Little Prince* (New York: Harcourt, Brace, Jovanovich, Inc., 1971, p. 84).

I expect the unexpected. I swim below the surface of events. A useful plan for all of us who are inundated with admissions, with despair, with life: Keep what your heart has learned and handed you. Keep it in a poem.

TEMPLE DOG

Each dawn the dog finds it
more difficult to contort himself
into a reasonable imitation of his early days
when he was born a fierce bronze facsimile of himself
and set into place on temple steps by careful hands
during a celebration lasting days.

His thousand-year-old muscles and bones
aren't as supple as they once were
on that long-ago evening when lightning struck,
when he was left with the scariness of breath and
an angel reciting the rules of incarnation
while he longed for his empty head and sightless eyes.
Then the angel petted him. Her hand was rain
smelling of cedar clouds. Her touch was exotic
flowers offered by priests and barren women, flowers
retreating into petals blessing his cold paws
and bathing them with wilting heat.

He has learned to enjoy nights
racing wind into the mountains
devouring small willing animals
strolling incense-filled rooms where silent forms
loom in the shadows of glowing gratitude.

But it is days he likes best because children
through centuries of touching have rubbed his head
into a shining crown as they peer into his eyes
with the eyes of the angel. He feels his vast brass heart
beating with her words, "I am never far away,"
her promise that he is unaware his eyes give back
to the bowing children, his eyes meeting theirs
in an arc of air that hovers like radiant wings.

I've been in a poetry group that has met for an hour or so at 7:15 each Wednesday morning for the last seven years. We are a small, sacred circle of people who love words, and we're hooked on the creative process. Our poems come from words and phrases we write down in the first ten to fifteen minutes after we arrive and talk about what we've dreamed or done in the previous week or what's been in the news. Then we write for another fifteen to twenty minutes, wait in silence for every one to be finished, and begin to share our work. We continue to be amazed and strengthened by the way the words play in our minds and by the different images they evoke.

"Temple Dog" came from a statement one of the women made. She and her husband had taken in a stray dog, an Akita, that showed up at the church and was named Barney by the church staff. He loved the freedom of their country home and joyfully welcomed each visitor to their B&B. Return guests looked forward to seeing him. One evening, during a thunderstorm, Barney begged to be let in and huddled on the tiled floor in the living room (he knew better than to walk on the rug with muddy feet). As he softly whined, my friend said to him, "How can you be afraid, Barney? You're the temple dog."

I write poetry from moments such as these, when I feel the universe handing me an invitation, challenging me, or laughing and crying with me. I write to celebrate life, to save and savor it. I write because life's gifts can be brief, and because I want to remember as many as I can. I write at three in the morning, sitting in my backyard and listening to fluttering and crunching in my hedge. I write from dreams. I write from images of motionless doves on the leafless branches of my winter pecan trees in late afternoon as I watch the sun go down. I write listening to one of my granddaughters sing to her LEGO blocks as she builds shapes only she knows the meaning of.

I write to gain understanding. In *Writing the Australian Crawl: Views on the Writer's Vocation* (Ann Arbor: University of Michigan Press, 1974, p. 17), William Stafford wrote, "A writer is not so much someone who has something to say as he is someone who has found a process that will bring about new things he would not have thought of if he had not started to say them." He writes about the justification to put a word down. It's simple; do it because it occurs to you. I write to learn willingness, to be receptive to the words, the images, and the sounds that come. I write to play. I write poems because they let the language dance, let the language lead me into the foreign countries of my mind. I write to experience the healing power of poetry, the affirmation over and over again that I am a part of the universe, that, as a friend says, synchronicity lives. Our stories are connected, interwoven with language.

I write from words I scribble at work on my palm or on my census sheet, or sitting at that small table in the staff room filled with smells of salsa and fajitas left over from lunch, or in front of the computer where I'm entering data. Writing helps me balance losing myself in the tumble of admissions, codes, charting, and wondering whether my job will be downsized tomorrow. Writing waits in the secret places of my heart for my return.

To me, writing poetry is like a cool drink of water after running a race on a hot day. I believe so strongly in the healing power of poetry that I became a certified poetry therapist, which means I use not only poetry, but journals and other literature to help people access feelings, memories, and events on a deeper level. A poem is powerful because of the language it elicits from the writer, the surprise. A poem contains both metaphor and paradox. Opposite feelings exist in the same sentence; this juxtaposition allows new insights and increased awareness. Through metaphors, we describe emotions and actions in new ways, which allows us distance and perspective. The page is nonjudgmental. We don't have to worry about commas or about choosing the "right" word. We can speak our hearts.

In his pioneering work, *Opening Up: The Healing Power of Confiding in Others* (New York: William Morrow, 1990, pp. 46–49), James Pennebaker studied the effects of writing about traumatic situations. He asked students to write for twenty minutes on four consecutive days about traumatic events in their lives, often events they'd never told anyone, such as sexual abuse, suicide attempts, and feelings of guilt. In comparison, other students were asked to write about superficial topics such as describing a room. Each group had blood samples drawn on the first and last days of writing, as well as six weeks later. Dr. Pennebaker found that students who wrote about traumatic events had enhanced immune-system responses. They sought health services less often over the next few months than they had before they wrote, and significantly less than those who wrote about superficial topics.

John Fox, a certified poetry therapist, (interviewed at Stephen F. Austin University, Nacogdoches, Texas, in 1998), compares writing a poem to how our immune systems operate: "I feel that the words and voice of a poem—the act of writing, of working on words so they say what one means, and the way that the words work upon us—is similar to the response of our immune sytems to a wound or a disease, an action to maintain wholeness and encourage optimum well-being."

We nurses are witnesses to life. Sometimes that's a joy, sometimes a sorrow. When we write poetry and share it with others, healthy things can happen. Expression of the feelings contained in the poem often moves from venting and/or labeling into communicating on a deeper level. We can let others see us. Scared. Vulnerable. Seeking healing. We learn that others are with us in the same trenches. They can say "yes." They can disagree. And we don't have to defend ourselves. Affirmation comes from putting our words, our voices, on the page and being heard.

Though I wrote "Temple Dog" more than a year ago, I didn't see until the writing of this commentary what a metaphor the poem is for my writing journey. In stanza one, the phrase "facsimile of himself" seemed relevant to the many years I didn't write. Then, at midlife the opportunity arose that I'd longed for. Could I do it? Did I have anything to say? Like the temple dog, I was "left with the scariness of breath," longing for the safety of my "empty head and sightless eyes."

Things changed when "the angel petted him." I began to hear my own voice. Stories and poems spilled onto the page like "exotic flowers." The whole tenor of the poem changes here, with images and textures layered upon each other. The more I accepted that the process of writing was truly a gift from outside myself, from The Creative One, I too "learned to enjoy nights / racing wind into the mountains," though I felt the shadowy side of life galloping beside me; for without shadow, how do we know light? The line "devouring small willing animals" surprised me. I tried to take it out, and it wouldn't go. I asked it what it wanted, what it meant. I remembered that Native Americans often thanked the animals they hunted for their willingness to feed them. I felt gratitude to the language that fed me.

In the last stanza, I write of touching, an act that has always been powerful for me. The children touched the dog, "rubbed his head / into a shining crown." Not a crown of material success, but rather one of successfully giving back the gifts we have been given. We do not know who will teach us, who will remind us, by a look or by a word, of something we once knew and have forgotten. Something about ourselves we must acknowledge and share.

I've watched the movie *Field of Dreams* countless times. I am always touched when Shoeless Joe Jackson, standing on the baseball field that Ray Kinsella built because he heard the voice, talks about "the thrill of the grass." I promised the muse that when she called I would be ready with pen and paper. The thrill of the words—when they invite me into their sensuous arms, I dance.

SUNRISE

In this canyon
where prayers of centuries
rush like wind,
I greet the dawn.
In the wash,
water sings
its careful song
over old footsteps.

Cottonwood and Russian Olive trees
exhale silent green light.
The sun begins its slow smile
down red canyon walls.
Broken trees raise arthritic
limbs in supplication.

Benevolent eyes
in the canyon wall
remind me I am loved
by this earth—my mother.
In this stillness
my breath blesses me.

But robins cannot keep quiet.
Nor can I.
In the motions of an old dance
my feet move like silk across red sand,
my hands posture gratitude, and I bow.
An orange and black beetle
crawls my prayer away
into the bones of the canyon.

I wrote this poem in Canyon de Chelly within a week after the death of my mother at the age of 97 in May 2000. Mom had died in a nursing home where she'd been for the last sixteen months, in a town where we had lived together for more than five years. I was in Albuquerque for a National Association for Poetry Therapy meeting where I received certification as a poetry therapist. After the conference, I planned to go on to Canyon de Chelly for a week-long poem-making camping trip led by John Fox. It was to be my reward to myself for persevering for several years to complete the certified poetry therapist requirements.

My decision to attend the meeting, though Mom would be in the capable hands of nursing home and hospice staff, had been difficult and surprising, the most recent in a long trail of similar decisions. It had been a journey in which my anger and hers were transformed into compassion, a journey during which we became closer. Though I had decided to go, I hesitated to leave her. For days I had packed, unpacked, and lain awake at night, wondering if she would be alive when I returned and thinking I had some kind of control over what might happen.

On the Sunday before the meeting began on Wednesday, the Sunday when I had to say yea or nay, I spent the afternoon with her. She was reclining in bed, sometimes dozing, sometimes picking unseen things from the air with her veined, arthritic hands, and sometimes talking about her sisters and brothers who had gone before her, wanting and not wanting to follow. In previous weeks, we'd had several conversations in which she spoke of the good life she'd had, and that now she wanted to go "home, truly home." I told her I loved her and would miss her, but I knew she was tired and told her that I, too, wished she could go truly home. As she dozed just before supper, I rolled back and forth in her wheelchair, rocking myself and letting my mind wander as I watched the setting sun through the blinds.

When I looked back at her, she was awake and looking at me. I reminded her where I was going the next day and why. I still hear her words: "I wish you wouldn't go." But what my body heard was "GO!" It felt like a blow to my stomach, and I rolled back in the chair. I don't remember what I said, but I was filled with the presence of this dual conversation with our words and with our bodies. Poetry reminds me, always, of this duality, this paradox, these conflicting feelings. I have learned to listen to incoming messages and to act upon what I believe to be true. When I left Mom after supper, I returned home to finish packing.

On my way out of town the next morning, I stopped to see her. She'd been bathed and was tucked into bed with blankets all around her. We hugged good-bye and she closed her eyes. She appeared peaceful and small as I looked back at her from the door.

I had attended national conferences of the NAPT for more than ten years. I knew the conference would be a swirl of speakers, workshops, and contacts with old friends. The workshop content varied. Always, we had a chance to learn more about and experience the healing ways of poetry and journaling. We also had many movement workshops. To me, writing poems is intensely physical; learning ways to use my body to listen, rest, and access my creativity was important.

The four days in Albuquerque were long, emotional, and informative. I called the nursing home daily. Mom was holding her own. On Thursday, the hospice nurse said she was "chipper." That word surprised me; Mom hadn't been chipper in years. In retrospect, of course, I think it was an outer manifestation of the inner decision she'd communicated to me when I last saw her. She was, finally, ready to go.

By Saturday afternoon, I was restless and tired, and my neck hurt. The last workshop I attended was about body-centered therapy, which teaches that the body is a source of wisdom, that the core of the self is inside the tissues, and that the body knows how to express the feelings contained there. The workshop leader invited us to move about the room, let our bodies speak to us and take us where we needed to go, and then write about it.

Initially, I tried going to my neck, but it was silent. Suddenly, my hands began to tingle, and for the next fifteen minutes they did a dance of their own—fingers wriggling, swooping, clutching, making fists and shadows on the wall, flapping like wings, running a gamut of emotions. I couldn't wait to pick up the pen and write about what my hands were telling me.

After writing, we talked about what different parts of the body represented. Hands have to do with letting go.

Twelve hours later, Sunday morning at 4:43 A.M., I received a call from the hospice nurse telling me she'd been with Mom when she'd died just moments before. "Your mother died beautifully," she said. I didn't have to ask what that meant. She'd died without fear. She'd died knowing she was loved and either hadn't wanted me there or wanted to spare me seeing her die.

As the conference wrapped up that morning, I was comforted by friends who hugged me and handed me tissues to dry my tears. I was in exactly the right place. My close friends back home were out of town. My children didn't live near me. That morning spent writing and being touched by the people of the poem-making community soothed me.

I was struck by the incredible timing of Mom's death on the very day the meeting was to end, the day I'd planned to return home instead of going to Canyon de Chelly. It meant that I had a choice. Mom and I had made her funeral arrangements long before she went into the nursing home. We'd even written her obituary. She was to be cremated and returned to Michigan to be buried next to my dad. After long talks with my children on the phone, I decided to go on to the canyon.

It was the right choice.

The canyon nurtured me with its space and with its subtle colors of light and stone. Our group of fifteen were wonderful companions. We wrote poems together, walked and climbed together, and I had time to go alone to a cave or a wash or to sit in the sun near a prickly pear cactus where Mom seemed to be particularly present in the orange and yellow blooms. The canyon walls and rock outcroppings invited my imagination. Opposite our campground, halfway into the canyon, the layers of rock looked like a face watching me with benevolent eyes as though, from a nearby place, Mom still looked out for me.

I heard again her voice telling our family stories. Evening stories told by our Navajo hosts around the campfire (you must have a Navajo host to enter Canyon de Chelly) told of the long line of people who had come before and those who would come after. Their myths. How they lived. And what they believed about death. They believe that when a person dies, he or she returns to the earth, to dust, to life again in trees, corn, or other gifts from the earth. The Navajo respect everything. I was comforted by the respect I felt for Mom's life. And for my own. I was comforted by thoughts of my grandparents and my grandchildren. And by the sounds of my family myths dancing and sizzling in the flames beside ancient myths shaped by stars traveling overhead.

Rock art deepened my feeling of belonging, of being in the right place. Particularly the white and red painted handprints on canyon walls and hard-to-reach places, such as the high ceilings of caves. A cautious climber and a victim of vertigo, I wondered how a person could climb up fifteen feet to leave a handprint overhead. I got dizzy thinking of it. I knew why a person would want to. To say, "I was here. Remember me." So much of Mom's and my relationship revolved around our hands.

For me, "Sunrise" contains all the images surrounding the story of Mom's death; "Water sings / its careful song / over old footsteps," the "slow smile" of the sun, "Arthritic / limbs in supplication."

"Benevolent eyes . . . remind me I am loved / by this earth—my mother." Place gives structure to memory, to story.

We hold our stories in our hands while we are alive, and when urged, or when we think of it, we write them down in poems or paragraphs for those who come after. If we die leaving them unspoken, then others come upon only parts of them in drawers where yellowed white gloves lie or in clay casts of small hands made in kindergarten. Or on canyon walls and in caves where the wind taunts us with whispers from the past.

I had been given a week of grace, a place where poems waited to be born so they could work their magical, healing power on me. Poems I wrote about the canyon and about my place in it for that brief time helped me name my feelings—gratitude, anger, sadness, love, joy, acceptance, hope. Not that I ended my grief work in Canyon de Chelly. I began it.

I started writing when I was eight. I wrote a four-line, rhymed poem about a sailor home from the sea. Maybe it was a past-life experience. I believe we have past lives. I believe that the healing work I do with language arrives from another time. I am grateful for the opportunity to do it again in this life.

I keep writing because of the joy and the surprises—the "Oh!" of recognition when I take up the pen. The chance that someone else may say "Oh!" when he or she reads one of my poems, which, of course, I will rarely know. And, more importantly, the chance to give back some of the creative spirit that's been given to me and to restore it to the earth and to ill people in need of that spirit. Life hands us rare and precious opportunities. As nurses, we get more than our share, and I am grateful.

Poetry Publications

Mercer's poetry publications include the following books:

Compassionate Witness: Before We Say Good-bye. Fredericksburg, Tex.: Barons Creek Press, 2005.
No Limits but Light. Chapbook. San Antonio, Tex.: Chili Verde, 1994.

Mercer has poems published in the following journals:

American Journal of Nursing; Icarus; Kalliope; Negative Capability; New Texas; RiverSedge; Wild Turkey; Windhover.

Mercer's poetry is included in the following anthologies:

Between the Heartbeats: Poetry and Prose by Nurses. Ed. Cortney Davis and Judy Schaefer. Iowa City: Univ. of Iowa Press, 1995.
Threads of Experience. Ed. Sandra Martz. Watsonville, Calif.: Papier Mache, 1996.
Women and Death, 108 American Poets. Ed. Jesse of the Genesee and Dorian Arana. Ann Arbor, Mich.: Ground Torpedo, 1994.

Mercer has contributed poetry to the following text:

The Healing Environment Without and Within. Ed. Deborah Kirklin and Ruth
   Richardson. London, England: Royal College of Physicians of London,
   2003.

Mary Jane Nealon

✿

Nealon confesses in her poem "The Priesthood" that she is "a keeper of things that don't belong to me." Ping! The clear ring of truth! She "keeps" patients, stories, memories, and more by preserving them in poems that are rich in metaphor and symbol. According to Nealon, "everyone must have a story," and those she "tells" in poems, wrought with the skill of a true wordsmith, show that Nealon is a "caregiver" in every sense of the word. She is a witness, an acute and responsible observer with all senses on alert. Walk softly in the cool dense forest of her metaphors.

I AM WALKING THE RIVER trail along the Clark Fork, thinking of patients. Melting snow has raised the river, so the coots with their black and gray bodies bob like nuns on white-capped waves. From the spindle of a dead tree, a bald eagle peers then dives down, wide and uninhibited in its search for food. The eagle is a poet flying into the raging water. Sometimes I dive down like that, onto an idea, into a phrase, and rise up, my mouth full of sustenance, but more often I am the heavy-bottomed coot, bobbing like those Weebles-wobble-but-they-don't-fall-down toys from when I was a child. This search for balance, for the life that sees and tells, for the energy of the poem that comes from witnessing, is all around me and carries me.

I am trying to remember when I decided to live in this river. I was eleven. It was summer in Avon-by-the-Sea, New Jersey. My father bought me an extraordinary spiral notebook, with five sections of colored paper: blue, pink, mint green, yellow, purple. "Here, do something with this," he said. I don't know if I decided to write a poem because I'd just read *Hiawatha*, or because it was the year that all the girls in my class decided not to talk to me, or because I was sunburned and confined to the shade of the porch, but I took the pad and wrote the alphabet out across the top of each page, then composed rhyming verse all day. I remember everything about that day, my legs pulled up under me, the sway of the wicker rocker, and the concrete planter with red geraniums.

It was a gate unlocked. It was a bay window wide open over crocuses in the grass. It was a *Naked Ape* of a day.

My father was a cop and a subscriber of beauty, so I have always understood the way the two lives meshed: the hard edge of homicide photos in an FBI newsletter and the swirl of paint in the books with art slides he ordered each month by mail. My father, Captain of the Renaissance. He would call us to the parlor, still in his uniform, and read the paragraphs about each painting to us as we fidgeted on the couch. "This here is Degas' 'Woman at the Bath,'" he'd say.

One day, when I was twelve, my brother and I were burying toy soldiers in our tiny backyard when, two doors down, the Polish man's collie started barking and jumping at the fence. Then we heard a woman scream. My father appeared from nowhere and leapt the fence; we followed after him, already bored with summer and making little funerals. The Polish man had hung himself in his shed, and my father, in one movement, pulled a knife from his back pocket and cut him down. He leaned over him and breathed for him. I remember the wife keeling and crying. I remember the black and white police car—the *Mickey Mouse,* we called it. The man survived, but his voice box had been crushed, so he never spoke again. He would glare at us when we tried to pet his dog. "He's never forgiven your father," my mother would say. But I saw my father after that as a kind of superhero. I started reading biographies, looking for the kind of life I might have, some way that I might be a hero as well. I read books about Kateri Tekawitha, Clara Barton, and Molly Pitcher.

I think everyone must have a story, or a moment in time that defines him or her. Mine is my brother's death from cancer. When he was diagnosed, I had already decided I wanted to be a nurse. My aunt, who lived with us until she got married later in life, was a nurse. I loved the extreme whiteness of her uniform. I admired the way she would stop at a neighbor's house to check a dressing after surgery, or the way she would sit next to the chair of someone in pain, lean forward, and touch them. I was in nursing school, standing at the nurses' station and watching my instructor demonstrate giving an injection, when our family doctor came and took me aside. "I'm not sure what this is with your brother," he said, "but I think it's bad." I knew at that moment my entire life was changing. I was holding a clipboard and little index cards with lists of medicines. I remember looking down the hall, seeing all the doorways, and understanding how each room had a story like mine. Some bad news had come on a beautiful day and changed everything for them, too. I felt connected to all the people in those rooms. Comrades. Secret prisoners.

I think now someone might have talked me out of what I did next: I got a job in the cancer center where my brother was being treated. I rationalized my decision by saying he was in pediatrics and I was on an adult floor. Of course, I was on a *young adult* floor, and many of my patients were just a year or two older than my brother. I had a hospital apartment across the street, so the last few months of my brother's life, I could work, see him, run home and sleep, then work and see him again. He told me many things in the months before he died, but most importantly he taught me a way to be with someone who was young and dying. I lost any fear I had about the bedside. I lost all fear of the suffering body.

In those months when he was wasting away, when his bones announced their sharp edges, I was reading Rilke's *Duino Elegies* and writing poems about my brother. I started to develop this habit of watching the body for little clues. In Rilke's Eighth Elegy he says something about looking outward like the animals, and I noticed that in their suffering poses, so many of my patients seemed to be staring out, looking for what might come next. I stopped challenging the Catholic Church and bypassed churches all together. I watched people nearly leap from their skins into the afterlife. I became convinced that the shift I saw on their faces as they edged from living in the body to not living in the body as a kind of moving into wisdom. Almost every person I saw die took on a physical peace. Their bodies seemed to lengthen.

So there I was, twenty-two years old when my brother died, living in New York, and reading poems. I kept a little journal about the things I saw in the hospital; most of the stories made it into bad poetry, and then I was through with it. The practice was its own ritual: work, pay attention, write it down, move on. But occasionally a person or an image or a story stayed with me and I couldn't find a place for it to live. "Human-Headed Bull below Empty Space" tells such a story. I never knew why the sight of the girl in radiology was so crucial to my life, but I knew it was; after my father died, I understood its importance.

HUMAN-HEADED BULL BELOW EMPTY SPACE

I.
On the lapis cylinders from 2900 B.C. images of the domestic
and the wild wrestle demons and musical instruments.
A human-headed bull braces a dulcimer while a bear plays and a fox
nestles at their feet. From *my* life, one scene inscribed
like that, so for twenty years a girl appears and reappears
in dreams. I am a young nurse, crisp uniform, high polished shoes,
carrying specimens that must be dropped off, when,

in the late after-hours of a cancer center, I get turned around.
I am lost somewhere in radiology. In each darkened room, huge
machinery and radioactive danger signs. Just minutes before,
on the ward where I worked, I massaged the feet of a boy
with testicular cancer. I rubbed his arch, and on a sketch pad
he drew my hands with charcoal. Precise lines he smeared
with his thumb. *You know, I just thought I was bigger
than the other boys in gym class,* he said, and added his own feet
to the drawing of my hands. Now the night has stopped itself
in this hall, and in my memory of him, the air is all enormous
cathedral. I turn left, and see a girl, whose back is to me,
standing before the new ultra-modern scanner, alone, arms outstretched,
her blue-and-white striped hospital robe, too large for her shoulders,
has fallen, and her hair, which I know will soon fall out, is luscious
and just barely reaches her hip. I watch her for how beautiful she is,
for how faithful she is to her position there, her arms held exactly,
for how she could be anyone, for how she could be me. The technician
arrives, directs me, directs her, and I resume the pace of someone found.
Some nights I dream I am photographing her, or painting her. And now
that I have seen the treasures of Ur, I dream I am carving her body
onto a lapis cylinder, then roll her onto parchment.
She is my link to a moment still before me in my life, before
I had cleaned the body of my father, newly dead. A moment in which
who I am is variable. I might have been the bear making music,
or the obedient human-headed bull supporting heavy strings.
But I have been frozen again. Mesmerized by my father's freckled skin,
as I turn him to place below him a clean sheet,
one the funeral workers can take with them. I love the way his vacant mouth
accepts his false teeth, I touch the black sores on both heels,
and the yellow, tobacco stained nails of his right hand.
I carve the sight of him on my retina, roll him
across my cornea, his arms, like hers, once reaching out, now folded.
And I know, because I have never forgotten *her,* that this moment with him will last,
just the two of us, in the middle of the night, before I call anyone
to help. I sit down for a while, slide my hand under his, and watch.

II.
Because now I have raised her up. Because now I have laid him down.
I tell her story to a friend who writes.
Maybe he will want to take her, and I will be able to let go
the responsibility of her fate, which has tracked me through the years

like a lion. Or the boy, whose testicular tumor
grew to incorporate his brain. Instead, my friend tells me *his* vision:
a night when he watched a dog from his city window.
Framed by the building's edge and the alley's long line,
light from an unknown source, moon, maybe streetlight, this dog,
curled, was reduced to *form,* his head and tail equal and still.
He remembers. I remember. The dog as girl as my father as a boy
as witness. Obedience and repose. My father *is* a dog a girl a boy
a human-headed bull falling below empty space, and it occurs to me,
that it is *this* which held us, *this* is what haunts, how we both saw,
for a moment, the empty space we are destined to fall through.

This is a poem that came from a culmination of stories collected over my years as a nurse, and from an understanding that no matter how good we are with establishing boundaries with our patients, their stories influence our lives. My father always tried to prepare me for the unexpected. As a policeman, he had seen ordinary days turn into a catastrophes many times. He was always warning me about other people, about unseen dangers. He and I talked once in the car while he was driving me from the airport in the pouring rain. I told him I was having nightmares about this girl I'd taken care of in New Mexico whose leg had been amputated at the hip. I told him I'd had to press my own gauze-wrapped fist against the hemorrhaging in her hip socket while they got the OR ready. I didn't understand the nightmares. I had written a poem about her. Why wasn't that enough? His response was to park the car in the storm and tell me about a car accident he'd seen as a rookie cop. The passenger had been unrestrained, and when the car hit the side of a truck, the passenger went through the windshield and then slammed back down into the seat. The passenger's head landed outside the windshield on the hood of the car and spun around to face its own split body. My father said he had failed to understand that it was his job to protect the driver, to get him away from the scene, so when the driver, an old man, turned to the passenger to see if he was all right, he saw the neck, and then the head on the hood, and died from fright. I realized in that moment that I could tell my father anything. I never dreamed about that girl again.

RAPTURE

*

On the rocks this morning an elephant seal gives birth. Blue head and smashing
    pink fluid.
Everything begins in violence, a bystander says.
The autistic says, *waves, there's waves, there's lots and lots of waves.*

*

I held an eleven-year-old girl in my arms. The hospital had bad linoleum, curled
    and sharp. We were in a ten-bed ward, stench
of old blood and afterbirth.
The girl, raped in the Duncan Projects, described being upside
      down on the metal stairs, and a ripping.
I held her as she gave birth to his baby: a stillborn with two heads—
one tiny undeveloped head arising from the neck of the true baby.

*

My father saw a crime in everybody.
Suspicion was a kind of wildflower for him.

*

My brother said he saw Jesus before he died,
but then again, he was trying to find ways to reassure us.

*

I saw a boy in New Mexico.
I saw him on a gurney and he was stunningly
handsome; the back of his head had been shot away
and it was my job to keep it packed with gauze
while we waited for his family to say *yes*
to his heart, his kidneys, his skin.

*

Sometimes when we make love
and I am upside down in bed
or I am cupping your head in my lap,
I remember the girl with the baby,
I remember the handsome boy.

*

My father told me that once, on Brunswick Street, a freight train headed for
    Secaucus
crashed and a bull broke free.
It ran past the Lorillard Shoe Factory, past Tony's vegetable stand and Juan's
bodega. It crushed Mr. Capezolli's roses, and then turned on the street filling
with people, and raced towards Monk Donoghue's mother, and speared her
against a car.

You have to be prepared for things you could never imagine,
my father said. But remember, suspicion was a wildflower for him,
was a beautiful weapon against surprise.

*

When my brother's heart monitor went flat
Jesus was a greeting card in the room.
My father was unwavering in a blue sweater; I thrust
my face into the wool of it. He was *immovable,*
but he had been preparing his whole life for catastrophe.

*

My friends sometimes ask me to tell stories about people dying.
I've never seen anyone die badly, I tell them.
Everyone is always peaceful, I say.
The autistic says, *waves, there's waves, there's lots and lots of waves.*

I always loved the phrase *ministering to the sick.* I miss the old days as a nurse, before the heightened technology, when my job was to give backrubs, pass out juice, and change sheets. Nurses aren't smarter now than they were then—we applied the chemistry and physiology and pharmacology we knew, but we did it with fewer machines; we relied more on our ability to read the human body. Spending time with the body helped me understand who was dehydrated, who was septic. My instincts were honed, sharp as a knife. I relied on touch, the feel of the skin, its heat, its clamminess. Being a poet also helped me learn how to see small details about a person. I was always paying attention. In some ways this made the work more painful.

I remember a man in San Antonio—I'll call him Raymond. He was fifty-two years old and dying of pancreatic cancer. He had a wife, a four-foot-eleven-inch bundle of energy with blazing red hair, manicured hands, and a series of sweaters she wore over her shoulders with little clips, the old-fashioned kind: two poodles, two ducks. One day, his children brought in a slide projector and sat with him in the dark, showing him their lives. He was turned on his side, and as he watched the pictures of himself hoisting his children in the air or pulling his son in a red wagon, I adjusted his morphine and wiped up the blood that oozed continuously from his rectum. I remember feeling so honored to be there, the click of the slide projector showing his life, and that life now leaving him quietly from his rectum. I had a hand on his back and could feel each beat as his heart sped up from the shock of losing so much blood. I remember feeling more like a priest than a nurse, more like a witness than a caregiver.

THE PRIESTHOOD

I

I thought I'd be a priest
or an Indian Saint like Kateri Tekawitha—
she survived small pox with blinded eyes and a disfigured face.
The book about her was the first thing I stole.

I took a chunk of fudge and gave it to my brother.
I wanted to be *heroic*. Caught,
I was forced to tell Father Griffith, but in the confessional,
I wanted to be the powerful one, not the sinner on the other side.
I made a private vow.

Pope Paul the VI appeared on the steps of St. Pat's.
The crowd screened, swooned.
Blessings flew in the air. I thought I was seeing Jesus
and nearly fainted from hysteria.
My mother pointed to the Pope,
he's just a priest, she said to calm me.

I wanted to *be* a priest: person in charge of ceremony,
magician of body and blood,
absolver of thieves like me.

My brother discovered a tumor. *Grape fruit*
they said. As though a tangy comparison could calm us.
I stole many things that year: the useless scapula
on my brother's bedpost. Fishnet stockings.
A change purse: small and green and leather
with a hammered rose. My stealing embarrassed the family.

Every Wednesday I was sent to after-school confession
for bad kids and adulterous wives. My priest idols
tilted their heads towards me,
whispering delicious forgivenesses.

Remember, my mother told me, *a priest is just a man.*
When my brother was nineteen, God suddenly swirled
in the invisible, an *idea.*

My mother's hand lingered on my back at my brother's deathbed.
She turned away from the final moment.
Everyone but us in the hallway when the clotted blood left his pelvis,
flew from the nest of his beloved lower belly,
and traveled to his heart. There in the room above the river,
he stared at me, breathless and afraid. His ribs,
like the hull of a boat, bowed out. And I in my fantasy
laid my hand on his forehead and told him how to go.
Convinced him of the way to go. Blessed him with my secret
priestness. Between us, the idea of God took shape.
This skin-to-skin pressure in the face of death's fluent body.
My mother's hand to my back while she looked out the window.

II
Before my mother died
she lifted her arms so fast
she hit me in the face.
She was trying to *throw* her arms around me,
did throw them,
heavy as they were for her
who could no longer lift them.

When she did die, at 3 in the morning, I had fallen asleep,
my head on her knees, her hand on my head.
All the others were in their rooms, restless or dreaming.
I woke to her breath giving out, woke to her hands reclaiming my brother,
to her turning back from the window in the room where he had died,
turning finally to face him. And I left them there.
My hand on his forehead, her hand on my hair.
I am a keeper of things that don't belong to me.

The truth is, the Jesuits brought small pox to the Indians.
They brought the need for conversion: fear
in the face of the epidemic. And Kateri Tekawitha,
scarred and made unbeautiful, wanted to be near them. Knew
that they would touch her, as they touched all the disfigured
and unpure, just as I knew
that the clap of the priest's incense holder released more
than the musky scent of God.

Kateri Teckewitha used to minister to Indians with smallpox, and she developed terrible scars that disappeared at the moment of her death. "The Priesthood" is about her selflessness and how the idea of being *blessed* entered my life. I know now that it was the grandiose imaginings of a child that led me to believe that nurse, saint, and priest were somehow one and the same. The miraculous thing was that it was this false idea, this mixture of story and myth, that allowed me to be with those I loved when they died. I am grateful to all the patients in my life who taught me how to be a guest at death.

I've always believed that we invite others to join us in every ritual—christenings, birthdays, weddings, baby showers—and that we also invite people to our deaths. Every bedside I've been allowed to be at, every death I have been blessed to attend, was at some unspoken invitation. I had managed the pain medicine correctly, or touched the suffering one with just enough respect, or brought water at just the right time, and my reward was to watch the miracle of the passing, of the opening to the next unknown.

And yet I am sometimes tired of helping people. I turned out not to be a saint or a priest. I have always dreamed of a life where I would be able to just read poetry, write it, and talk to people about it. I resent the way the day can disappear in the ordinary tasks of helping others. The predictability of the day. I work with people with HIV/AIDS, and have for many years. Once there was a terrible energy about how catastrophic it was for those who were diagnosed with AIDS. Tragedy has its own energy. I was in a frenzy of writing poetry, trying to respond to this unknown epidemic, to the frightening changes in the bodies I cared for: large sarcoma lesions and swollen limbs, dementia, wasting, and intractable diarrhea.

I remember calling an undertaker with a patient who was trying to make his own funeral arrangements. He was a musician and had beautiful hands. We made the arrangements and then he sat in his wheelchair and leaned forward and put his head on my shoulder. I remember my blouse was wet with his tears. "I feel like I am living in a Kafka novel," he said. On the way back to his room we marveled at the exotic flowers in the lobby. "Look," he said, "how they change everything." I remember the fear before we knew how AIDS spread, and I remember touching people despite the fear.

Now my job has become more about *entitlements* and *benefits* and *housing assistance*. I feel sometimes like a veteran, home from the war, asked to provide maintenance to the tanks and jeeps.

Poetry remains a kind of sustenance, like bread. "Who Dies of Thirst" comes from the sense that I have lost time, that days with poetry disappear somehow more quickly, more fully, than days without. It asks the question that I struggle with: if I am not a nurse, if I am not a caregiver, what is the value of my life? All the questions I have for life, all the questions I have for poetry, are answered at the bedside: at the birth of a newborn or at a death. Sometimes, though, I just want the joy of the day and to shrug off all the images I remember from twenty-eight years of nursing.

My parents used to come to my poetry readings and my father continued to come after my mother died. What changed in the experience was that, before my mother's death, my father functioned like an undercover agent at my readings. He'd go out for a cigarette afterward and say, "What did you think of that girl? The nurse?" He'd then report to me all the little comments he could gather. After my mother died he would come and cry during the reading. A silent, dignified weeping. Poetry was a way for us to talk to one another. After he died I found a poem I'd written for him years ago, laminated and face up in his bedside drawer. I remember friends saying to me, knowing how close I was to my father, "When your father dies you're going to have to be hospital-ized in a loony bin." Instead, everything I learned from nursing, everything I learned from poetry, became a way for me to let him go. Just days before his death I told him I wanted him to try some morphine. "No, Mare," he said. "I don't want to be too sleepy. I want to see how I handle it, and I want to see how you handle it."

It was like that day in the storm in the car when I told him about my nightmares and he told me about his. All fear went away, and we were sitting together in a beautiful storm.

WHO DIES OF THIRST

*

On my desk the dahlia is a fisted door
is a feather falling between myself and the man I am trying to help:
train-jumper, *transient*. After three days in the Thompson Falls jail
his body's rancid scent overwhelms me. He is a criminal trespasser.

I go with an escort to his trailer, which straddles a ravine.
The rusted shell explodes with mice, attracts
a red-winged hawk. The sky a berth behind the circling
hawk, I escape for a moment in the wing's spiked tip.
We leave medicines, lift the wire fence back in place.

I latch the day. Across the road a spitting llama
rolls in pink flowers. Inside, in my gut, a cramp
of what I no longer want to give away.
I am tired of serving people.

*

I believed I would live like Kateri Tekawitha.
Disfigured, she leaned over the parched lips of Indians,
caught in their blistering small pox.

I would rise every day into *goodness,* place
cool cloths on foreheads, make pumices
and plasters, and then at death,
like her, my scars would rapturously fade.

I would ascend, luminescent.
This was the wildflower story I was living in.

But my back gave out from lifting bodies in their beds,
from leaning over the colostomy's rosy stoma.
I resented the way people held on to me, in labor,
in death. I saw birth as a *tearing away* of flesh.
I carried my imagined *real life* in a metal cart strapped
to my ankles. Everywhere I looked: faces,
when all I wanted was the empty desert.
Red rock of the free life.
Carved wall of the vacant cave.
I ate delicious words when I was alone.
What will I be if I am not a caretaker? My hands
are flat expressions of themselves, are unrecognizable.

*

This morning, an explosion of gnats and flies,
sweet maple window
drawing them to *this* life, as I am drawn to leave mine.
I call in sick
and fall into Salmon Lake
which has become a kind of room where green
is nothing more than a cool cool day.
Lake, open and rocky, my hands are returned to me

as they pass over lily pads and shift the silt
that coats dark water. The floating leaves are words,
words are bubbles that rise to the surface
circling my thighs. Words smell like pine.

*

The lake is a velvet confessional,
I kneel in its arms. The lake is thought, and memory.
In the water, my dead brother rises, clean of agony,
and we are watching art slides after school
with my father. Our knees touch in the dark
as we practice dry, innocent kisses on our hands.
The lake is the gold parlor of my childhood.
The lake is a book. The lake is my first lover,
my best lover. The lake is the moon we thought we would colonize.
The lake is the colony we named Lorca.

In the distance a siren heads down Highway 83,
and the sound of a child falling sounds like a child
falling away. The day moves from east to west over water.

Can I be left in my cool lake?
Can I *be* the cool lake?

I eat a slice of apple; I eat a slice of pear. The juice of the melon puddles on
the plate. NPR plays opera. It is a Saturday in Montana. The locals argue about
the wolf's reintroduction to Nine Mile; the Cosmic Cones Little League team
giggles under my window on their way across the field. I read a translation of
Baudelaire by Ciaran Carson. Baudelaire sounds like he is in an Irish pub. Just
as I finish, my seventy-one-year-old cousin calls from Ireland. The world is
serendipitous. And luscious with blooming lilac. My neighbor has a band; they
play Santana's *Oye Como Va* better every day. I turn off NPR and listen to them.
Two squirrels sit, asses together on my ledge, looking in opposite directions.
I remember the Bowery and the man named Eddie who drew chalk drawings
of the god Janus on his flophouse wall and made penny sculptures and cried
when he talked about his melanoma. "I smell like I'm already dead in places,"
he said. And it was true—he was putrid and gangrenous, but I didn't mind
being near him because his eyes were crystalline blue and he had made these
drawings of the god Janus and sculptures from pennies. He doesn't yet live
in a poem of mine, but I want him to. I want to slay the monster of his flesh

and let him go over the Clark Fork to rise and fall over the rapids under the shadow of the eagle.

My friend is working on a poem about death. It is a sonnet of seven couplets. She wrestles so much truth into two lines that I am breathless. We hear breaking news about a Painted Lady butterfly migration. They are coming from Utah because of El Nino. They fly at the height of a small child's head. So many are killed on the interstate that the road is closed in places because their dead bodies have made driving too slick. The poem is like that. Hovering in its gentle opening and closing, and also part of a current so powerful, it circles the globe and changes the temperature of oceans. The poem, like the butterfly, lives among us, at the height of a seven-year-old. We sometimes lie on the grass to see it from the underside, and sometimes, in our haste to get past thoughtfulness, we run it down and slide in our heavy bodies over it and away from it. But what an act of creation! I believe nursing allows for witness, and with that witnessing comes responsibility. Poetry carries the energy of story. Poetry is dependable. Poetry begins with a small word, a thought; poetry flies on air currents across deserts, over broken rivers, over snow-capped mountains in June, and down into the valley to sit beside me faithfully this day and every day.

POETRY PUBLICATIONS

Nealon's poetry publications include the following books:

Immaculate Fuel. New York: Four Way Books, 2004.
Rogue Apostle. New York: Four Way Books, 2001.

Nealon has poems published in the following journals:

Forklift Ohio; Hanging Loose; Heliotrope; Kenyon Review; Mid-American Review; Paris Review.

Nealon's poetry is included in the following anthology:

Things Shaped in Passing: "Poets for Life 2." Anthology of poets responding to AIDS. Ed. Michael Klein and Richard McCann. New York: Persea, 1997.

Geri Rosenzweig

Whether writing from the perspective of a "Flaxen God" or writing as her younger self, Rosenzweig pulls the reader into a new view of the world. Born in the midlands of Ireland, she knowingly describes a field waiting to be crossed as "patient," and this unique descriptor leads the reader to a deeper contemplation of the fields from which human beings draw their sustenance. Because Rosenzweig is a nurse-writer, one can't help picking up on the double meaning of "patient" and "field." We tritely encourage "patience" in our sickest patients: take one day at a time. The bodies of patients, flesh and bones of our patient, are the "fields" in which we work; we create sterile "fields" for surgery and dressing changes. Throughout it all, Rosenzweig's poetry is intellectually provocative and bears the imprint of a faithful witness.

CROSSING THE FIELD

for Susan

We walked among the thin trees of December.
It was rural Ireland, small doorways,

silent fields, crunch of frozen grass
under our shoes. One of us said

I'll go to England, there's nothing here…
White plumes of our breath

rose as though in agreement, cities floated
distant as planets in the mind's sky.

The last field, patient as a shadow,
waited to be crossed;

they ran a highway through it years ago,
a line drawn through a paragraph of plans.

It was the sky darkening as we leaped
a ditch between field and road.

One of us looked back
at a landscape going up in smoke,

but it was only the light flaring
a moment on hills.

It was cold. No snow,
but the smell of snow, and no memory

of your hand in mine
as we touched ground.

WHAT MOVED ME TO WRITE this poem was a phone call from Ireland telling
me an old school friend had died of breast cancer. Almost immediately, the
memory of our walk across fields outside the town where we lived flooded
in. It was December, and I would be going to nursing school in England the
following spring. When you leave the place where you were born, everything
back there seems frozen in time—the landscape, the people. My friend and I
had been talking that day of leaving a place where, as the poem says, "there's
nothing here." We were seventeen and eager to run into the arms of the world,
a world outside the small, tight world of rural Ireland. The poem came rather
quickly as I remembered that, of the two of us, I was the one who left. If it's one
of my favorites, perhaps it's because of the way the language took over, without
too much struggle, which is always a gift for me; I usually work slowly, staring
at a blank page or up at the ceiling. I was pleased with the image of "the last
field" being "patient," which seemed to work off the impatience of the poem's
narrator to break away. Most people like the story it tells with its images of a
rural landscape; they identify with a young girl's eagerness to leave home.

I also like the line, "cities distant as planets." As a fifties' teenager in Ireland,
I was obsessed with the images of other places, cities especially, all that glit-
ter compared to a small town in the Irish midlands, with its one traffic light

and eternal rain! I found out much later that I'm happiest in so-called rural landscapes, close to nature; we always want the opposite of what we have. The poem ends with only one of us making it across the ditch, just as only one of us left Ireland. I wish I didn't have to write poems like this—I miss not having my friend in this world—but while writing it, she was with me in startling clarity, in what Czeslaw Milosz calls "the eternal moment."

THIS BACH CANTATA

Before shoes
lose the promise
of roads and coats
refuse the blare of sun,
before the comb,
crying for hair,
cracks its teeth
in the pantry
and the stove's
four rings glow
in the empty kitchen
while the kettle
sits on a chair,

before the children's
voices grow rough
on the phone,
O before I forget their names

let me remember
where the pills are,
the silk robe,
the carafe of wine.
Lead me to this Bach cantata
I put by with clear instructions.

Against morning
drifting light as a pair
of nuthatches to the feeder,
strengthen me.

This poem comes from the fear most of us have of growing old, of forgetting who we are, or where we are. I remember visiting my mother one summer when she was in her late eighties. I'll always carry the image of the four rings of the electric stove burning brightly as she sat at the kitchen table, reading the newspaper. Bright and cheerful as those rings were, I felt an emptiness run through me; I was losing my mother, this strong-willed woman who had been the center of my world for so long. Even her voice was getting lighter, and her eyes, once a deep green, were fading—she was fading from the world!

Poems tell the truth: old people do forget their children's names, and their children's voices do get rough with impatience. Of course, this poem is wishful thinking on my part; will I remember where I have put the pills when I reach old age? My friends and I have lots of laughs over the image of one of us standing in front of the fridge, trying to make sense of a note that says, "the pills and the Bach cantata are in the right hand drawer of the night table." Hmmm. The end of this poem is true for me—I love morning; it's the best time of the day—the light on the walls of the house, that feeling of beginning, everything new again. In the poem, I make plans for the end, but who knows. This life of ours is the only one we've got. I can't imagine forgetting my children's names, or leaving a comb in the pantry. Will I remember that I wrote this poem?

CALYPSO'S BAR

He's lost on the new coast road,
but the inn's a cave of light
and the barmaid is out of this world.
Her lilac hair is a sea rippling
on a summer's evening.
Her breasts glow like stars
in the net of her blouse.
She places a cold beer before him,
leans into his voice, a sound
she hasn't heard in centuries.
He plays out snapshots of home,
wife and kids, a ranch down south,
peach orchards, a golden Labrador in the yard.
Bright shapes glide between
willow and cypress in her fish tank.
She pulls another beer,
whispers words in his ear.

Her voice is wind rustling in a field of lovage.
He leans on the oak beam of her bar.
All night and years pass.
Her bed's phosphorescent with satin sheets.
He fingers the silver buckle on his belt.
The sea level rises.

I had been reading *The Wedding of Cadmus and Harmony* (by Roberto Calasso, translated from the Italian by Tim Parks, New York: NY, Knopf, 1993), a wonderful retelling of the Greek myths by Roberto Calasso. "Calypso" reached out to me with the writer's belief that one can find all of the characters in the Greek myths alive and well in our everyday lives; one can find a "Calypso" anywhere in the world in a bar late at night, and Odysseus too, a man leaning on her bar, probably a little drunk, and making a pass at her. Originally, the poem started with the line, "the barmaid is out of this world." I thought that sounded like a cliché, but in fact or myth, this barmaid was out of this world. I don't know where the last line came from, but it seems right—the "sea level" did get high for Odysseus that night. When I read this poem at poetry readings, it gets some laughs; people find the image of Odysseus as "that old goat!" amusing. We write poems about life, death, loss, grief. Most of my poems are dark, so when one comes skipping lightheartedly down the path, I grab it and have some fun.

PRISM

for E

Let your left hand rest
in the shadow of the soup bowl
while your right hand believes
in the spoon, and the spoon's hollow
rising to greet your lips.

If there's a window
where you are, let the prism
hanging there separate
the light, play its violet/yellow/green
ribbons over your face
in the long afternoons.

Let your slippers, obedient
as plush cats,
wait near the leg of the sofa,
let the visitor, hurrying
up the path, lift the latch
to find your hair grown back,
the wool cap you wore
flung useless in a closet,

then let me return to the world
in time to see the goldfinch
devour the heart of the cone flower,
crack open all the seeds at once.

Watching a friend fight the effects of a brain tumor, the effects of chemotherapy, as best she could, and cursing the wretched crablike cell which destroyed her life, I did what I could—I wrote a poem for her, or rather, the prism hanging in the living room window wrote it for me. The image of those colors playing across her face one day as I visited her will never leave me. Nor will the wool cap she wore, or her slippers by the sofa. She was diagnosed with cancer in the spring. As summer came around, I'd get back to my own house to find the finch on the cone flower; there was something about the way the bird gorged on those seeds, gorged on the fullness of its life, its unawareness of how sickness enters the body with no way for us to explain it. I must have about twenty drafts of this poem. It came slowly, and at times I did not want to work on it. I wanted to be off somewhere, maybe in another poem, or just shopping for my grandchildren.

If, as my friend believed, there's an afterlife, I hope a prism glows there. It's difficult to write a poem like this without that dreaded word "sentimentality" creeping into it. I hope I've avoided that.

FLAXEN GOD

Flax: found in the ruins
of Stone Age lake dwellings in Switzerland

My blue petals, open at sunrise,
    fallen by noon,
tell her it's time to lift me

from a rooted dream.
        I am stems crushed
under her stone.

My seed beds down
        in her wild hair.
But death is eased by her song

of what I become,
        something finer
than straw broken,

lowered into her pond
        where starlit water
frees me from a woody core.

When she gathers me
        into her arms once more,
lays me down to dry

in her field of light,
        I yield the long fiber of myself
to her rough comb.

Now I am all she desires,
        silken strands drawn
onto her spindle of bone.

 Recreated by her hands,
        woven about her hips
this spring, I enter the world.

This might be one of my favorites. Linen, that lovely cloth we all like to wear in
summer, comes from flax. After reading that flax had been found in Stone Age
lake dwellings in Switzerland, I had a wonderful time looking up the process
by which flax is turned into linen. I imagined a Stone Age woman working by
a lake, pounding the stems, the seeds flying into her hair. I was hoping to get
the whole process of linen making into the poem, without the poem sounding
like the directions on the back of a box.

In the first few drafts, the narrator of the poem was the woman, but it wasn't working for me. I put the poem aside for a while, then, as usual, when I was doing something else, the "voice" of the flax came through as a god entering the world each spring. After that, the language and content came together, like two people made for each other.

The verbs I used here—"raise," "crushed," "eased," "lowered," "yield," "woven"—describe, I hope, the process of turning flax into cloth, as well as the action of the flaxen god resurrected into the world each spring. I wish I knew the reasons for why I write. I suppose I write to make sense of the world, to make sense of my own life. I write because I want to, because I've always been in love with the language of poetry, with metaphor, image, the cadence of poems. I'm never as free as when I'm writing. If it all comes together, I just look up at the ceiling and say "thank you!" The way a poem takes us down a path we know nothing of always knocks me out. Metaphor tells me what it is I'm trying to say, and how to say it. I often think of writing in terms of nursing—how nurses attend to people; poets do the same thing; we attend to the poem, waiting for it to tell us how it wants to come onto the page, when to leave it alone so it can get some sleep and do some serious dreaming; we take its temperature, give it some food, a back rub, a bed bath. Fanciful? Maybe, but so be it.

Nurses are witnesses. We do what writers do—we bring sounds into the world. Sometimes the sounds are cries of bliss, and other times they are cries of pain. When the poem seems finished, if a poem is ever finished, we pronounce it well enough to go home, home being somewhere out there in the world of poetry journals, book publishers, or just a friend's letter box or e-mail.

One of the meanings of the word "imagination" is "the power to form mental images of things not seen before." Since poetry is a point of entry into the buried life of feelings, imagination is the engine driving my writing. It brings up the past and restores it to the present. For a while, I'm in a timeless place, groping for words after the first impulse of the poem has knocked on the door. Imagination looks for ways to enlarge our everyday language through simile, metaphor, and rhythm. Imagination is attentive. It notices things while the rest of the mind is busy with making coffee or writing the bills. It holds images, thoughts, and ripples of sound until we're ready to give ourselves to the writing, give ourselves to what haunted the ear and mind long before it arrived on the tongue. Have my literary skills made me a better nurse? Actually, it might be the other way around. Being a nurse made me, I hope, a better writer. I go back to that word, "attentive." I was attentive as a nurse; I'm attentive to the poem. When language, rhythm, and syntax work together, there is a feeling of completeness, of bliss. That lasts for all of five minutes! Then I want to write the next poem.

POETRY PUBLICATIONS

Rosenzweig's poetry publications include the following books:

God Is Not Talking. Johnstown, Ohio: Pudding House, 2002.
Half the Story. Greensboro, N.C.: March St., 1997.
Under the Jasmine Moon. London, Ontario: HMS, 1992.

Rosenzweig has poems published in the following journals:

Antigonish Review; BBC Wildlife Magazine ; Cape Rock; Confrontation; Greensboro Review; Natural Bridge; Nebraska Review; Nimrod; Pearl; Poet Lore; Poetry International; River City; Sulphur River Literary Review; Verse; Voices Israel.

Rosenzweig's poetry is included in the following anthologies:

Anthology of Magazine Verse and Yearbook of American Poetry, 1995–1996. Ed. Alan F. Pater. Palm Springs, Calif.: Monitor, 1995–96.
Intensive Care: More Poetry and Prose by Nurses. Ed. Cortney Davis and Judy Schaefer. Iowa City: Univ. of Iowa Press, 2003.
Life on the Line. Ed. Sue Walker and Rosalyn Roffman. Mobile, Ala.: Negative Capability, 1990.
The Next Parish Over: Irish-American Writing. Ed. Patricia Monaghan. Minneapolis: New Rivers, 1993.

Paula Sergi

ℰᶈ

In her poem "Lake de Neveu," Sergi describes leaving nursing for a career where she "swam / in blue ink." Fortunately for us as readers, she weaves an informative tale of her personal journey, revealing the power of nurses' narratives to make sense of a chaotic and painful world. Furthermore, her words demonstrate the power of language to artfully link her two careers so that each empowers the other. As the other nurse-poets in this book make clear, the two careers are not separate at all. Overcoming the nurse's challenge of "locating the authority to speak," Sergi advances her readers toward the empowerment inherent in the use of codes and language.

SINCE 1992 MY WORK HAS focused on language. I've been a working poet, an editor, a student of writing and, most recently, a writing instructor. Occasionally my background in nursing becomes a topic of conversation, usually through my own reference. My former career is unique among my colleagues, and I feel a mix of pride and wistful regret at the work I did as I came into adulthood. At times I miss the rigors of the scientific method, the illusion that there are answers to our questions that are either correct or incorrect, either supported with evidence or not. As Louise Glück writes, "It is relatively easy to say that truth is the aim or heart of poetry, but it is harder to say how it is recognized or made. We know it first, as readers, by its result, by the sudden rush of wonder and awe and terror" (Proofs and Theories. New Jersey: Ecco, 1994, p. 34).

I'm often asked how I shifted from a career in nursing to one in writing. Once, when asked this by a poet friend, I tried to describe my years working in home health. I began by saying, "It isn't that I didn't want to touch them." My friend was astonished with the phrase, and she challenged me to write a poem beginning with that line. The resulting poem is "Home Visits," and though the triggering line was later shifted, it remains the emotional center of the piece. Merely suggesting that a nurse would hesitate to touch her patients hints at a truth recognized, as Louise Glück suggests, by "the sudden rush of wonder and awe and terror." It is that line that struck my friend Kate, that makes readers uncomfortable, and that made writing the poem so important to me.

HOME VISITS

No wonder I paused at their doorsteps,
measuring the distance between us:
my shining young skin, my white teeth, white shoes,
my crisp jacket, new job, fresh breath.
Before the knock I'd hesitate, checking their charts
for the wound where the pressure of time
had worn holes in their skins.

Most were near the end of their unpeeling,
shedding layers of memory and money.
On the other side of their doors, the acrid
ammonia of urine melted in their bedding,
their trousers and stockings. Drainage-soaked
gauzes trailed behind as they shuffled
to answer the bell.

I wrote *care* plans directing my visits,
mapping the way those wounds would heal,
from the outside in, and listed what I'd use
to fill them: ointments and creams,
plastic sheets like skin itself glued over
their oozing gaps. Orange-colored scrubs
or vinegar. Even sugar sprinkled on like faith.

With my little healer's tools I listened to the pressure
of blood against their vessels as their corpuscles tried
to escape. Catheters drained their amber urine
and plugged up and had to be plumbed. Urine bags
hung like handbags over walkers or bed rails.
I poured their pills into plastic cups, marking
time on calendars big as their kitchen tables.

But I was distracted: the corners of their homes,
the cobwebs and cuckoo clocks, veneered end tables,
scratched woodwork, what the windowsill

figurines could say. Sometimes I'd hear about
lovely mothers, the children they never saw again.
And when the hour was up, I'd shout
my instructions and leave.

It's not that I didn't want to touch them.
We had no idea, back then, about age
passing itself on. It's taken years
for me to recognize a skin that won't
bounce back, a stuttered gait on icy walks,
elusive words that hide behind
the floaters in my eyes. Once in a while

I'd see it when I washed their bony backs,
a used-up body about to lift off
with scapular wings. The glitter of dust motes
above their bird-like heads as they sat
by their windows watching me coming
and going, still lives of another kind. Above
little cloud-tufts of hair, haloes for the almost dead.

This poem represents the emotional core of my transition from nursing to writing. As the details of the work come back to me, so does the memory of my fascination with my patients' homes and lives. The fourth stanza makes reference to my distraction with details beyond my job duties, with "the corners of their homes, / the cobwebs and cuckoo clocks, veneered end tables, / scratched woodwork, [and] what the windowsill / figurines could say." As the poem suggests, I became interested in the stories behind these details and spent time imagining what I could not know. Because of my nursing education in skilled observation, I was able to make note of the many physical details that comprise a character's life, and I found myself wanting to record and expand on these details, to explore, develop and fictionalize these realities. The process of story-making, of course, helps to contain the sadness and suffering nurses confront in their daily work. Molding the details into a narrative or a tale helps temper the realities of illness and the inevitability of death. For me as a nurse-poet, imagination becomes a way to escape the difficult realities of aging, the illnesses and loneliness so prevalent among the elderly.

The poem also hints at a sense of futility in dealing with the chronic nature of my elderly patients. I remember deliberately illustrating that feeling when I made reference to "my little healer's tools." By describing the stethoscope in diminutive terms, I gave voice to the frustration of dealing with the certain deterioration of elderly patients. Of course their healing is slow; medications only manage the symptoms of advancing cardiac failure and of progressive chronic disease.

Because so much of the home-health nurse's work involves maintenance, after a couple of years as a staff nurse I moved away from direct patient care and into a middle-management position. I was ready for different challenges. Ah, the impatience of youth! Had I known then that the situation of nursing presents a uniquely rich opportunity to observe human nature, I would still be working in home health. Where else can a person be welcomed into another's home, invited to sample their favorite recipes, encouraged to look at their family photographs, and privileged to hear about a person's life stories and personal philosophy? My experiences with the Visiting Nurse Association had as much to do with my becoming a poet as my lifelong interest in language. By looking at how I came to write "Home Visits," I can identify that the success of the poem has to do with my ability to address both the strengths and vulnerabilities involved with nursing. This becomes particularly clear when I consider another of my poems about the topic.

On Switching from Nursing to English

Losing the white nursing shoes was easy—
they made my size eights go on forever,
boats that said too much,
defied the fashion rules for Labor Day,
and Easter.
Dumping the uniform was good for self-identity.
I don't miss the contact with bodily fluids,
and I feel nauseous less frequently in class.

But, as any student of the English language will say,
the problem is the spelling.
Grimm did not explain the sudden shift from *b* to *v*
and I write *bowel* all the time.
Come to think of it, no bowel shift allows for what happens
to the *e* from *pleural* and I think *pleurisy, effusion,*

a plethora of problems with the lung, over and over, to indicate
more than just once. Confusion reigns longer
than William, and I attribute it

to the influence of French.
These days I'm better dressed, but
where am I headed with a longer,
misspelled resume?

Looking over this poem, I see how it skirts emotional truth by making light of
the surface differences between my two careers, the spellings and misspellings
of words, the costume or uniform, playing with the issue of identity. There's
no attempt to confront the complex questions that are behind such a dramatic
life change. That's not to say that there's no place in life for more light-hearted
fare. But the essence of poetry is its ability to touch different people in differ-
ent ways by its language, its form, and, of course, its truth. As a nurse-writer,
I sometimes struggle with the process of telling the truth behind the issues
I confront. I usually find it when I reach the visceral core of an issue, and
this is treated lightheartedly in the "Switching" poem. In contrast, there is
much body-centered language and imagery in the following poem about my
childhood.

FOUR ON A FOLD

Some summer night in the early sixties
in the middle of the country,
no ocean for miles
in either direction, the air was everywhere heavy
like grandma's mothballed wool quilt,
navy as night
covering our faces, holding us down.
We should've been tired from play;
four square, seven steps around the house,
hopscotch drawn from the sharp side of a stone
on squares of concrete that marked
the edge of our lawn.
Those nights we could stay up till nine,
but even after sunset no air moved.
We'd try to sleep
in the ten-by-twelve family room,
windows on three sides,
as if the screens themselves
would make a breeze.

Four on a fold-down couch
in short polyester pajamas that stuck
to our backs waited for sleep,
for a breeze, for a father
who never came back to say good-bye.
I worried maybe we'd all suffocate
before dawn, but we all grew up
one way or another
before we realized how little air we'd had.

In this poem, I consciously selected sounds to mirror the heavy sense of loss I felt when I lost my father at the age of three.

The oppressive heat of summer in the Midwest is described with the slow sound of the phrase "no air moved." The seemingly hopeless reality of discovering that the presence of screens themselves could not make a breeze reflects a child's ability to give up on magical thinking in favor of reality. Here we find children who "waited for sleep, / for a breeze, for a father / who never came back to say good-bye." I've received a lot of feedback about this line; I think it is a favorite with audiences. I imagine that the emphasis of sound in the poem is the absence of a father and the absence of a breeze. The holding of one's breath, really, is felt by the audience. On the other hand, there is the absence of air, with a play on words in the absence of the father who creates an "heir."

Can a writer be true to the experience of childhood? In my observation, the careful selection of detail helps pin down the elusiveness of memory. The poet can leap from what is remembered to imagine more details that help to give an arch or shape to the poem. In this poem, the specific aroma of my grandmother's quilt led me to other memories: the games we played, the sidewalk itself, the limits placed on us by our mother. These details naturally led me to recover the area of perceived rules about being a child in the 1950s. The physical limits of the sidewalk, the lines and boundaries of four square and hopscotch, help to reinforce this notion.

In turn, these limitations remind me of other expectations for my child-self. For me and my siblings, there were no discussions of grief, no school counselors, and no family therapy sessions. After my father died, we simply went on with our lives, trying to ignore the huge void and its implications. Because such a loss has emotional ripples that continue to affect me today, my father is a subject that I return to again and again. It is as though I can recreate the story at whim, and revise the endings, such as in the following poem.

LAKE DE NEVEU

We could only swim by invitation and one came
finally via mother's second husband
after he left and the step in-laws felt guilty
for the wide wake of his drinking.

In my ribbed swim cap with the yellow water lily.
In my sister's faded suit, too long in the body.
I wondered how a lake could be called private. Was it
because this one was deep, with secret seaweed

way below?—unlike the stagnant public Winnebago
beach, no more than a marsh bed of pond weed,
cattail, bull rush, a breeding place for warty frogs.
When I surfaced from my shallow dive,

always the careful child, I imagined I swam
in blue ink. I drew circles on the lake's clear face,
writing stories of a long ago carriage lost
as it skirted this lake's wooded edge, slipped in

and was swallowed, no trace of horse hoof or bridle
ever found. A cloud on the surface mirrored
heaven where my real father sat on a cumulus couch
holding his halo and my kindergarten drawings of a family.

Tiny waves fluttered like the ruffled borders
of a photo circa 1955, father still here,
departure whispering from the corners of his smile.
Maybe the fairy of glacier lakes dives into de Neveu

taking father number two in trade. Bubbles from silver bass
brushed my ankles and I waited for my father
to emerge from the lake bed, from the shoulders
of the lost men, from their horses' slippery backs.

Though the child in this poem still waits for her father's return, she takes
control; the act of imagining another scenario helps her to deal with the loss.
Making a story about the carriage's disappearance both illustrates the depth

of loss and gives it a location. The child also locates the father in a physical place. Though heaven is illustrated as an intangible cloud, a halo (at least in the form of a grade-school angel costume) is a palpable item. This child has also illustrated her wish for a complete family through her "kindergarten drawings," and in imagining this action the adult writer reaches for resolution. The whole idea of death is very "slippery," but the use of the word, the availability of imagination, and manipulation of retrieved memory make the act of writing therapeutic.

Writing this poem also led me to see how my father's death left his family without a social status. When he was alive, we were clearly a lower-middle-class family. But when the head of the household is eliminated, where are his survivors left? We were clearly public-beach kids, and a flirt with the upper class, however brief, was confusing. It added to the emotional complexities of my childhood. Writing the poem helped me to sort through those issues.

The experience of being a mother also presents a writer with creative challenges and rewards. The call of mothering and of writing create a struggle to locate the time, the justification, and the words to accurately describe the experience. The two worlds seem entirely separate, mutually exclusive, because they require such different skills. Naturally, great tension builds in the mother-writer.

GERMINATION

—*Gray's Manual of Botany*

Firstborn, the day you cracked into the world,
dark hair, olive head, unfamiliar yellow face,
not at all the blonde baby my mother had,
I wondered what it meant to hurt this way.
Your alien almond eyes never closed,
The nurses had never seen a newborn so alert.
You searched all things foreign, all things not me,
turned away my breast, my lap, my lullabies of boats
that sail away, come back, sail away.
I thought I sang you gone.
You learned too young to break restraint,
constant sunstrain, craving everything beyond our door.
My heart split with the yoke of every day,
While the world chanted *cross, jump, climb.*

Now, your sudden need to shun morning,
avoid chinks of light, meet friends
at night in bowling alleys,
lean toward those with small, dark homes,
gravitate to their green and gold
broken down sofas, breathe smoky basement air.
In this, your second birth,
I step over your wet towels left on the bathroom floor,
watch your silent, lurking growth,
wait for you to shoot
into the dark luck of teens.

In 1985 I became a mother for the first time at the age of thirty-two. Though I should have known better with my age and experience as a registered nurse, I was shocked at my newborn's homely features. Despite what I'd learned from school and in ten years of public health, I'd somehow expected that, after eighteen hours of labor, I'd be holding a replica of my baby picture, the one hanging in my mother's bedroom where I, at eighteen months, was rosy cheeked and dumpling cuddly. Here he was, born two weeks late and showing all the signs of a post-term baby. Dry, sagging elephant skin hung around his skinny legs. At just over five pounds, he most resembled my foreign-born father-in-law.

After just twenty-four hours in the hospital, I came home to care for my newborn. Sitting in the rocking chair in the freshly painted nursery, I held him and sobbed as I acknowledged the certain pain involved with loving someone beyond reason. At that moment I was simultaneously aware of our sudden attachment and already entangled in the process of letting him go, imagining the day he would no longer need me and would walk away from the home I would spend eighteen years creating for him. Some people would nod and acknowledge postpartum depression, a biochemical reaction. But I know that my experience that day with my newborn was nothing short of a vision. Perhaps this is when I first recognized the intuitive power in a relationship involving a close physical bond. Much has been written about women writers' unique connection with the body and spirituality.

Though I had been writing seriously since 1992, I avoided writing about my children until entering an MFA program in 1999. My hesitation had to do with the fear of creating poetry that fails to express the truth about being a mother. The subject seemed too risky, the potential pitfalls of sentimentality too great. I worried about the value assigned to a poem on such a domestic subject and whether I could be true to this complicated topic. And, what if my mother or husband should see such a poem? What about my son, and the fragile peace we negotiate on a daily basis?

When I wrote these lines about my son, revealing my reaction to his physical appearance and that he felt like a foreigner to me, I felt guilty about having and expressing those thoughts. It seemed contrary to what I'd learned about mother-infant bonding. Yet I knew I had come upon some essential truth in my writing, and that sensation was exhilarating. It felt dangerous to say that this infant seemed "alien," improper to describe him as "foreign." Yet it also felt liberating. As I proceeded to explore this emotional territory, I discovered a related sense of personal responsibility for his early independence—certainly my "negative" thoughts somehow created his risk-taking behaviors during his adolescence. This ambivalence toward myself as a mother led me to the emotional center of the poem, embodied in the lines "I thought I sang you gone."

What, then, do my poems about losing my father and being a mother have to do with being a nurse-writer? By looking carefully at my work, I've noticed a pattern in the way my lines and poems develop. Writing about motherhood suggests a split between my domestic and artistic self, just as writing about my father highlights the chasm and proximity between the vulnerable child and my adult self. There is something mysterious and wonderfully complex in these and in nurse-patient relationships, in the wonder over life itself and the tenuous thread between life and death. These are situations that demand impossible love and disciplined distance, a confusing palette of both positive and negative emotions that surprise and confound the writer. My experience as a mother-writer involves a split between my domestic and artistic selves. Being a mother means being organized and practical, yet constantly emotionally available. The demands of nursing seem remarkably similar.

For the nurse-writer such a split involves equally complicated questions. Nursing requires one to be available at all hours for both highly emotional interaction and simultaneous highly skilled tasks. A nurse must be humble enough to consider the input of other health-care professionals, gentle enough to be compassionate and nonjudgmental, yet brave enough to inflict the pain inherent in treatments and procedures.

Another area of conflict for the nurse-writer is the tension between the nurse's watchful eye and the poet's faithful recording of the emotional interpretation. Though keen observation is central to both roles, the kind of detail required in writing poetry can become complicated in the realm of patient confidentiality. A nurse-writer's job is to expose the truth, which might include writing about her own honest reaction to a patient, a procedure, or a diagnosis. Through exposing her emotional pain and the related range of feelings, she may be exposing her patients in a way the nurse-professional would never do. Confronting and describing this kind of work presents a challenge and an emotional journey.

As a serious nurse-writer, I know I must confront a difficult situation. Can I find the aesthetic distance necessary to write a poem about other peoples' misery? Will such writing trigger an automatic, negative response from readers jaded by the confessional nature of such poems? Is there any value assigned to this writing? Can I be true to the topic, with its complicated associations with joy, despair, guilt, and vulnerability? What about the grip of confidentiality?

Locating the authority to speak presents yet another challenge. Cultural norms have propagated the myth of the nurse as subservient and silent. As Alicia Ostriker notes in *Stealing the Language* (Boston: Beacon Press, 1986, p. 180), women writers such as Adrienne Rich demonstrated that what we have is a flat and sanitized version of the mother-child relationship, which is "institutionally useful but experimentally inauthentic." We can make the same claim about the role of the nurse in our culture and in literature. Despite Cherry Ames's dedication and cleverness, wasn't she really always under the influence of Dr. Joseph Fortune? One need only glance at the covers of nurse-romance paperbacks for assurance that the most a nurse can hope for is to be the object of a male physician's lust. This bit of fiction masks the rich give-and-take which characterizes relationships between the nurse and physician and the nurse and patient.

Then there is the reality that caring for patients is centered on gender and flesh, a reality that has not always fit with the image and morals of a proper woman. In his widely circulated book, *Ethical Principles for the Character of a Nurse,* (Milwaukee, WI: Bruce Publishing, 1924, pp. 119–20). James Brogan cautioned student nurses:

> If all the physicians and surgeons were saints, if the intern and the staff doctor and the family physician were above reproach, the nurse would still have need for prudence and guarded conduct and a modest reserve. You must nurse married men and young men. You must be with them alone through the long hours of the day and night. Your kindness and attention will by their very nature cause a certain attachment. In the beginning it may be only a natural gratitude and perfectly proper. Here comes the danger: for this feeling grows, and before either party is fully aware, there has sprung up an affection.

And we all know where that can lead. Though Mr. Brogan puts some blame on the nature of male physicians, it is the female nurse who is held accountable. Happily, our culture has moved beyond these cultural stereotypes, but the shadow of such ingrained thinking lingers and complicates the nurse's role.

I expect that the emerging, authentic writing by nurses will *continue* to break these stereotypes and demonstrate that we are no longer willing to romanticize the role. Nor will we conform to what previously might have been considered "poetic" or "acceptable" writing. The energy in writing by nurses lies in the intuitive counterpoint to the reams of objective data that we are trained to collect and record. Nurse-writers provide the counterpoint to the conventional medical model. By seeing beyond the body, making connections and projections, and filling in the details with an artist's eye, we have opportunities to illustrate what can't otherwise be known about patients and ourselves. The act of caring provides us with a unique range of human emotion from which to write.

I look forward to more nurses speaking honestly about the unique and challenging situations we face. With nursing currently under a microscope, such writing will illuminate the profession's complex role and draw attention to the many significant issues currently under consideration to address the nursing shortage. In the hands of competent writers, the current challenges in health care will be examined and the drama of human experience well recorded. The complications that challenge us will help us illustrate with an unflinching eye.

As Louise Glück (*Proofs and Theories,* p. 54) reminds us, "When the force and misery of compulsion are missing, when the scar is missing, the ambivalence which seeks, in the self, responsibility...when ambivalence towards the self is missing the written creation, no matter how artful, forfeits emotional authority." As nurse-writers we have a unique opportunity to confront our actions, admit our fears, and address the split between our strengths and our vulnerabilities.

POETRY PUBLICATIONS

Sergi's poetry publications include the following books:

Brother. Fund du Loc, Wis.: Action, 1996.
Family Business. Georgetown, Ky: Finishing Line Press, 2005

Sergi has poems published in the following journals:

American Journal of Nursing; Bellowing Ark; Bellevue Literary Review; Black Dirt; Blueline Press; Crab Orchard Review; Crania; Farmer's Market; Fox Cry; Inky Blue; Manzinita; Mediphors; MM Review; Potpourri; Primavera; Rain City Review; Rattlewind; Rosebud; Slipstream; Small Pond; Sow's Ear Poetry Review; Spoon River Poetry Journal; Wisconsin Review

Sergi's poetry is included in the following anthologies:

Boomer Girls: Poems by Women from the Baby Boomer Generation. Ed. Pamela Gemin and Paula Sergi. Iowa City: Univ. of Iowa Press, 1999.

Climate Controlled. Ed. Alder Monson. Grand Rapids, Mich.: Diagram, 2001. http://www.thediagram.com.

Fire in the Womb: Mothers and Creativity. Ed. Elizabeth Anderson and Kate Smith-Hanssen. Philadelphia: Xlibris, 2003.

Intensive Care: More Poetry and Prose by Nurses. Ed. Cortney Davis and Judy Schaefer. Iowa City: Univ. of Iowa Press, 2003.

Kelly Sievers

❧

Sievers writes with graceful ease about holding on and letting go. In her poetry we see the merging of the art of words, music, and museum and cafe graphics—and nursing. The poem "I Dream Gene Kelly Is My Father," based on the narrator's dream on her wedding eve, illustrates the power and longevity of family narratives. The oral history in this instance is a romantic once-upon-a-time story of a father being mistaken for "the nation's romantic hero." Such mysterious narratives have long and multiple lives, as seen in this talented daughter's poetry. The poetic and literary precision of Sievers's work echoes the clicking steps of an elegant dancer—and of a nurse anesthetist. There is art in the dance, in the words, and in the nurse.

HOLDING ON

Twenty-five years of airports between us, we still part
as mother and child. I watch you press
your purse to your chest as my plane pulls
onto the runway. You wait, guarding
your vision of me, until nothing holds
your eye and clouds christen us separate.

You say ticket counters are no place to separate,
follow me to the gate and do your part.
I never tell you I need time to hold
a roll call for my divided selves, to press
myself whole again, always guarding
against letting your laugh, your hands, pull

on the short line that divides us. I pull
from your stories now to separate
the mother from the woman. You guard
the romances, tell of January swims, parts
of childhood dares: toppling outhouses; pressing
friends to hide in attics, skipping school; holding

prohibition parties. The stories hold
a vision of a father's daughter, pulled
to echo his love of football, cigarettes, pressed
to stay at home, "College is not for girls." Separation
came in pieces: a '33 Plymouth, Chicago, New York. Parts
I played, thirty years later. And what of the guarded

line to your mother, a woman whose past guarded
a son? I've heard you ask, "What takes hold
of a woman to leave her child, so much a part
of her?" You told me how you pulled
her past from Aunt Kate: first marriage, separation.
I remember Thanksgivings when you pressed

your half-brother to join our family, pressing
out the wrinkles of difference, guarding
his bizarre, paranoid life. "Separated
from his mother," you'd say, "from any family to hold
onto." No family life to pull
from when he tried to play the part.

I left home at eighteen, pressed hard to break the hold,
always guarded against your pull.
I return now, separate, to be one of the parts.

MY EARLY POEMS EXPLORE FAMILY history and relationships. Both the content and title of this poem, "Holding On," reveal my struggle to establish an identity separate from the one bestowed by family bonds.

This poem was written between 1989 and 1990. I began searching for a creative outlet in writing classes in 1986. Poetry's compressed intensity and probing images were new and exciting to me. I also recognized writing as a means of exploring my life and relationships. In 1988 I took the class that would change my life. I began to study poetry with Floyd Skloot through the Oregon Writers' Workshop. Skloot is a widely published poet, essayist, and novelist. His latest book of poetry is *Approximately Paradise*. Floyd taught with humor and love; he nurtured us. I learned to compress words into truth. As I shaped my words and images, I began to see the shape of my life. I began to believe my words belonged in the world with all written words.

I searched for poets who wrote about family history and relationships. One of the first poets I was drawn to, Maxine Kumin, wrote her early poems in traditional forms. I discovered her as I made my way through the University of Michigan's Poets on Poetry series. She spoke of her process in *To Make a Prairie* (Ann Arbor, Mich.: University of Michigan Press, 1979, pp. 84–85): "In the early days we [Kumin and poet friend Anne Sexton] were both working quite strictly in form. We measured and cut and pasted and reworked arduously, with an intense sense of purpose, both of us believing in the rigors of form as a forcing agent, that the hardest truths would come right if they were hammered to fit."

By engaging me and the other students in an intense study of many poets, Skloot introduced us to formal and free verse poetry. In our studies, he revealed his love of formal poetry. His teachings reinforced what I had read in *To Make a Prairie*: the use of "formal patterns can render hard thought malleable, or at least bearable. Form can provide a staunch skeleton on which to set the flesh and blood of feeling" (p. 108).

The first text we used in the workshop was *Strong Measures: Contemporary American Poetry in Traditional Forms* (New York: Harper and Row, 1986). I learned that through rhyme and repetition, a poem's form could echo emotions and images. I was amazed and delighted. How perfect to "hammer" my recurring themes of separation and pull with my mother into a newly discovered form for me, the sestina. A sestina is a poetic form of six six-line stanzas with a three-line ending called an *envoi*. What an opportunity the length of the sestina provided for me to explore her history.

I carried the indelible image of my mother pressing a purse to her chest for a long time. The image was connected to life events. Around 1980 our parents moved to California from the Midwest to be close to my older brother and his family. A year later I began a new phase of married life in Oregon.

Travel between San Jose and Portland became frequent. Each time I left San Jose my mother insisted on a ritualized vigil at the airport. Although I appreciated the diligence of love implicit in every plane-waiting vigil, airport trips became painful. On one trip the airline, because of flight problems, transferred us to a bus for the San Francisco airport. As we pulled away from the curb I looked out the window. My parents waved from the curb, and my mother clutched her purse as if her entire life were in that purse, as if I were in that purse. I was nearly forty years old.

As I built image after image from memory to write this poem, I began to see the relationship I had with my mother from a new perspective. My relationship with my mother was a story. I wrote the story; I found my place in it.

I chose the end-line words for this sestina—part, press, pull, guard, separate—because they haunted me. The repetition of these words in the poem pulled me forward. When I reached the final three-line stanza, the *envoi,* the sestina-prescribed word pattern magically blended to give birth to the poem's ending. The sestina had led me to a discovery, to a bare-boned truth. Writing the final words, staying within the form like a dance step, gave me such a sense of freedom. I saw I could be separate and one of the parts at the same time, in the same life story. There was joy in that discovery.

I DREAM GENE KELLY IS MY FATHER

On the night before my wedding I dream
Gene Kelly is my father. The piano plays
"An American in Paris" and we are a team

leaping and gliding, Gene in his beret,
me in a tight black skirt slit to expose
one thigh. He lifts me, sets me on a café

tabletop. While Gene dances before
me I try to tell him my father does not wear
a beret; that he is a union man, worn

from too much overtime. If he danced
it was in the hours before my childhood
when he wore Ray-Ban sunglasses,

sent my mother a recording of
"I Don't Want to Walk Without You"
But Gene isn't listening. He holds

a rose up to me, I slide down into
his arms knowing this isn't right
my father and I are not this duo

but knowing I like
this slit skirt,
this father.

This poem, written a few years after "Holding On," represented a leap for me. My background—Catholic, blue-collar working class, sheltered—prepared me to follow rules, to write within the margins. In this poem I allowed words to leap from the actual story to a new, imagined place. I entered the world of risk taking through words.

The family tale that sparked this poem is one my father repeated through the years. In 1942 he became a civilian machinist at Pearl Harbor to help with cleanup and restoration. He traveled across the United States by train. Upon his arrival in Los Angeles, a woman approached him and asked, "Are you Gene Kelly?"

"No, I'm afraid not," he told her. She followed him a few paces. "You are Gene Kelly," she insisted. "I know you are. You can't fool me!"

If you squinted, my father remotely resembled Gene Kelly. He was a born hoofer and met my mother in a Wisconsin dance pavilion. Their romance, however, eluded me and my brothers. It remains their secret.

Many poems might have evolved from this family story. I could have written a poem, in my father's voice, inventing Hollywood capers. And what about my mother's dreams of capturing such fame and fortune? I focused on the bewilderment and awe this story stirred in me as a child. How was it possible that a woman saw my father as the nation's romantic hero, Gene Kelly? I stretched this wonderment into my adult life.

How to write such a poem? I began by recording the story and details (those Ray-Ban sunglasses!) in an abbreviated prose style. Then, days or weeks later, I compressed prose into "poem-length" lines. Reading and poetry workshops taught me the value of each word, which is the essence of poetry.

A syllable count of ten to twelve in the first few lines gave me a pattern. Somehow, three-line stanzas made rhyme easy and helped images flow. Using a rhyming dictionary, I played with off-rhymes. This invited new words into the poem.

I was surprised that the focus on my father exposed me to the possibilities of the romantic in him. Was it actually the process of writing that allowed this to happen? I think so. Writing poetry gave me a place to explore my imagination. The quiet hours I spent with words led me to wander down paths I did not know existed.

What gave me courage to take risks with words? Poems. The times I write the most poetry are the times I read the most poetry. I keep stacks of chapbooks and journals at my bedside, in the bathroom and the kitchen, and on the cocktail table. I discovered poetry as an adult. I must catch up. I never leave the house without a book in my purse. In Rich's Cigar and Magazine store, I read poetry crouched in a corner. Sweet pipe tobacco odors swirl in my nose; brave words fill my head. The men and women who put images and emotions on the page send me a message: "This matters."

ROCHESTER, MINNESOTA, 1965

Hot tunnels wound beneath the ground,
hospital to dormitory to chapel. But we

chose to run through icy
air. With stiff white wings pinned

to our heads, we hugged our breasts
and flew. From women draped

in long folds of white we learned
to pull back blankets, expose one

arm, one leg, to bathe
the sick. Here is the heart,

Sister Ruth said, showing us empty
chambers, valves held tight

on tiny strings. And the eye,
one big black cow's eye,

its crystalline vitreous
hidden. Beneath the light from

three-story windows we sat on gallery
benches to watch silent men

open the brain. At night
we dipped our fingers

in holy water then slid
into our single beds,

hiding our hot
and steaming hearts.

BIOPSY

She wants to know what time it is.
Did she sleep? She has no
time to lose in sleep since probing
fingers circling felt it nestled,

jewel-like, beneath her nipple.
A steamy mirror, one arm lifted,
stillness before words rose:
How much time? She needs to know.

Buttoning blouses, moving boxes,
turning toward her lover in
and out of bed, she feared it spoke
to all her cells in secret code
each hour, every stolen minute.

After I wrote a number of poems directly related to family, I opened my work life as a nurse anesthetist as a source of poetry. The process was slow. Early attempts to write about nursing were conceived and written in prose. An essay (*American Journal of Nursing*, Vol. 89, No. 5, May, 1989) melded a personal experience with surgery to reflections about patients in pain. The next piece began as a memoir.

Writing poetry was my creative outlet, an escape from the realities of hospital life. Therapeutic? Yes. I didn't know exactly how to shape hospital realities into poetry. I had not read any work by nurse-poets.

It seemed all my life I had been a nurse, and I wanted to be something else—a poet. As I became comfortable with poetry, I learned that poetic forms can embrace many subjects. The more I wrote, the more willing I was to expose "my nurse self" to the poetry world. A piece I began in a memoir-writing class turned into poetry because I didn't like the prose I had written. Too many words!

I worked hard to distill images for "Rochester, Minnesota, 1965." What Skloot taught us in class was evident: compression of words provides tension, and images gain significance. The reader becomes engaged.

My "memoir" became a poem. Writing the poem, and the way the poetry community embraced it, opened the way for me. Patients I met every day in surgery provided occasions for poetry. I was moved by the mysteries of their lives. Before I began writing poetry, I had no means to explore and appreciate that mystery. I also had no way to express my attempts to connect with their lives.

A woman who repeatedly asked the question, "What time is it?" as she awakened from anesthesia gave me the occasion for "Breast Biopsy." All of us know someone who has had breast cancer. Sometimes we know them well enough to know how it affected their lives. I was moved to imagine what this woman's life was like as she frantically repeated her question about time. Poetry gave me "the place" to imagine her life.

Does writing poetry affect the way I practice nursing? I don't know. I do know poetry gives me a medium to expand my vision of the patient, to see the "new" in daily routine. Writing poetry also places me in a realm of openness. I am more "present" in the world. Hopefully, all this makes me more available to patients.

IN THE HOUSE ACROSS THE STREET A BOY IS PLAYING A HORN

He is sitting on a kitchen chair, knees
parted. Sheets of music stand in a dresser
drawer. Pressing his lips to the mouthpiece,
he begins again. Over and over

he reaches above and below some note
he hopes to find. Then he finds
that note and rides it
to the ceiling. He leaves his room

where every night he lies in bed
waiting for the slam of a car door,
his father's stumble. He flies
from his house like his mother

flew three years ago, her coat
billowing behind her. The tip
of the boy's tongue pushes more notes
into the horn. Music

floats down the street.

When I am writing I am more precise and keenly present in the world. My observational skills are at their peak. At home, walking in the neighborhood, shopping at the market, I am more open to any experience, real or imagined.

Listening to the sounds of this boy's horn coming through my kitchen windows week after week, I began rooting for him. I began imagining his life. I didn't know why his mother had left him in that house. All I knew was that his horn sounds were a crazy mix of sadness and hope. How often we know only bits of information about people we see every day. Poetry gave me an opportunity to get as emotionally close to this boy as my imagination allowed.

I have read that we write poems to hold onto experiences, to images. Since the boy has grown and left home and I no longer live in that neighborhood, I am glad to have this poem. The piece you write becomes more the memory than the actual memory itself. It is like viewing photos of a vacation. Sometimes the photos become the vacation more than the events themselves. The memory of this boy is now tied more closely to this poem than to reality. That is okay. I like to think the emotional truth lingers.

Looking at the structure of "In the House across the Street a Boy Is Playing a Horn," I can guess that I began this poem by writing in rhymed quatrains. As I write drafts of poems, I read them aloud. Often more natural line breaks can be found that way. If the rhyme scheme doesn't fit the natural flow of the poem, I abandon it. A poem also has its own rhythm, established in the first line or two. In a *New York Times* review of *Dogs Bark, but the Caravan Rolls On: Observations, Then and Now* (Boston: Houghton Mifflin, 2003) by writer and musician Frank Conroy, the reviewer, Sven Birkerts said, "Finding the groove, in music as elsewhere, is never finally about proficiency—it is about trusting the rhythm of what happens and letting go into a deeper, more instinctive, if not truer, zone of the self." The more I write, the more I let go. I have learned to trust the rhythms of the poems I write, to trust myself. That's how writing changes one's life.

Outside the Hotel DeVille

"Le Baiser de l'Hotel de Ville, Paris, 1950," Robert Doisneau

He draws her close, gently presses her lips,
open, and she is lifted off the street. Isn't this
the kiss every woman wants? A thin dress
flutters at her knees. His neck scarf loosens
as he waves to the world with one arm.
In the crowd a man in a beret turns away,
a coarse-haired woman frowns.

Let her frown. Let autumn breezes ruffle
everyone's hair. Let jackets and sweaters
sail open. She has crossed the ocean for this.
She will paint scenes of pink nudes and purple
nights. She will float paper boats on summer
ponds, sing arias. One morning she will see
the light beneath her daughter's skin. One day
this kiss will make her plant red poppies
in the front yard.

A kiss like this could make
you walk up a stair, through a revolving
door, late for a date; late for an affair.
In the gilded lobby a man waves,
his suit jacket falls open. *You look
lovely,* he says, and reaches out.

I first saw a print of "Le Baiser de l'Hotel de Ville, Paris, 1950," a photograph by Robert Doisneau, in a neighborhood restaurant. I was enchanted. Who were these celebratory people? How did the artist, Doisneau, catch the intimate moment of the kiss? Did he know the couple? I had enjoyed viewing art of any form since my high school days when Sister Stephanie sent us to the university book store to buy *Gardner's Art Through the Ages.* The class was "Art Appreciation." To this day, whenever I ascend the wide steps of an art museum, a comforting calm comes over me.

Yes, Sister Stephanie taught me how to appreciate art. She also tried to teach us how to write about art. We would gather our notebooks, pens, and pencils and quietly enter the art galleries, wearing our gray school blazers and our starched white blouses. We described what we saw, compared it to what we had seen. I don't, however, ever remember pressing my imagination to dream about what I was viewing. Years later, poetry gave me the venue to do that. My notes for this poem read: *Let's say she's an American in Paris. It is 1950, the war has been over for five years. Anyone can sail to Europe. Believe that moment, that kiss, is the most important thing that ever happened to you.*

Clearly romantic musings! I may have been thinking about all those movies from the forties and fifties I watched on late-night television as a teenager. I could have been thinking about the three-month trip I made to Europe at age twenty-three.

In *The Writer on Her Work* (New York: Norton, 1980, p. 20) contributor Joan Didion wrote: "I write entirely to find out what I'm thinking, what I'm looking at, what I see and what it means." When I began writing in the early 1980s, Didion's words were my motto. Yes, I wrote to find out what I was thinking, but I clearly remember writing this poem because it was fun. I could write this poem because I allowed myself to dream. I count twelve drafts of this poem, but the middle stanza always stays the same. I wrote that stanza quickly, without letting my inner critic interfere. Entering that zone of freedom is like stepping into a dream.

The first time I realized that poetry could be written as a response to art or music, I was astonished. I knew poems of love and poems of nature. How wonderful to learn that I could write poems that would reflect on music and art, as well as tell history and probe relationships.

Sometimes I respond to a piece of art just as I might respond to someone I see on the street or to a patient who passes through my shift. Nurses understand this kinship. All those lives we witness every day. How could we not see, feel, the human chain of connection? Has writing poetry made me more open to the human condition? I hope so.

But I also know that I was a nurse first. I learned to give a bed bath when I was sixteen years old. I wrapped that washcloth around my hand, tucked the ends in, believing the person before me could be my mother, her friend, me. The art of nursing! My life was expanding in ways I couldn't understand. A writer must have a kinship with her subjects and empathy for the people she writes about. So must a nurse.

Poetry Publications

Sievers's poetry publications include the following book:

Making Room. Waldport, Ore.: Alsi, 1995. Winner of the 1995 Yachats Oregon
    Literary Festival Chapbook Competition.

Sievers has poems published in the following journals:

Bridge; Calapooya Collage; Descant; Ellipsis; Fireweed; Greensboro Review; Hayden's Ferry Review; HMS Beagle (an online bio-med journal); *Journal of Medical Humanities; Mediphors; Oregonian; Permanente Journal; Pittsburgh Quarterly; Poet and Critic; Poet Lore; Prairie Schooner; Seattle Review; Western Journal of Medicine; Writer's Forum.*

Sievers's poetry is included in the following anthologies:

Between the Heartbeats: Poetry and Prose by Nurses. Ed. Cortney Davis and Judy Schaefer. Iowa City: Univ. of Iowa Press, 1995.

Boomer Girls: Poems by Women from the Baby Boomer Generation. Ed. Pamela Gemin and Paula Sergi. Iowa City: Univ. of Iowa Press, 1999.

Generation to Generation. Ed. Sandra Martz and Shirley Coe. Watsonville, Calif.: Papier Mache, 1998.

Prairie Hearts. Ed. Whitney Scott. Crete, Ill.: Outrider, 1996.

The Soul of the Healer. Ed. Tom Janisse. Portland, Org.: Permanente Medical Group, 2005.

Kathleen Walsh Spencer

෫෬

Spencer demonstrates a willingness to play and experiment with form and per-sona, as she demonstrates in her pantoum "Coffee for One." The nursing process and the poetic process are similar in Spencer's estimation. Both require observa-tion, data collection, and a decision—an assessment and diagnosis—based on the data. Once a decision is made, a plan evolves—for the patient's care and for the poem. The form and structure chosen for the poem are important vehicles for carrying the poet's message. For example, stanzas, meter, rhyme, and metaphor structure the poem. Nursing standards, multiple local and national regulations, traditional protocol, and process structure nursing practice. Editing and revision are acts of evaluation and reassessment—writers and nurses cannot function without constant reassessment. Spencer describes, with a twist of humor, the process for the novice as well as for the experienced poet.

COFFEE FOR ONE

Sometimes I sing to see if my voice works.
In the morning, making coffee for one
I forget the omelet, make Pop-Tarts now.
Don't have to wait turns for the shower.

In the morning, making coffee for one,
I have the crosswords, sports and front page.
Don't have to wait turns for the shower.
I throw my wet towel on the bedspread.

I have the crosswords, sports and front page,
Read about terrorists, domestic abuse.
I throw my wet towel on the bedspread—
Hardly something to fight about.

I read about terrorists, domestic abuse.
Our sheets haven't been changed in six weeks—
Hardly something to fight about.
Her pillowcase smells like clover.

Our sheets haven't been changed in six weeks.
A crescent of lipstick rims a mug in the sink.
Her pillowcase smells like clover.
I take it to work in my briefcase.

A crescent of lipstick rims a mug in the sink,
Divorce decree on the countertop.
I take it to work in my briefcase.
Me-Me-Me, my voice squawks.

Divorce decree on the countertop,
Forget the omelet, I make Pop-Tarts now
Me-Me-Me, my voice squawks.
Sometimes I sing to see if my voice works.

THIS IS A PERSONA POEM. *Persona* is Greek for mask, and in a persona poem the writer pretends to be someone else. In this poem, the female poet takes on the persona of a recently divorced man. I had been stuck in a rut, writing mostly first-person narrative poems, that is, poems about my experiences. Well, that got boring, for me and the reader. I wanted to try different voices in my poetry, and the persona poem was a great way to stretch myself.

This poem was confusing for many readers (especially those who know me) because my name was on the poem, and the reader wasn't ready to believe that the "I" in the first line was a man. This may be why some poets just use their initials, like K. C. Spencer, to eliminate preconceived notions about the speaker in the poem.

Frequently, poets share their poems with other poets during the writing process in order to receive constructive feedback. This is often done in a group, referred to as a "workshop." Occasionally, a naive poet in the workshop will assume that a poem is true because of the "I" voice. I think people with backgrounds in the sciences are especially "guilty" of this because they live in a world of facts.

"Coffee for One" is also a pantoum. The pantoum is a poetic form with a prescribed pattern of repeating lines. The second and fourth lines of each four-line stanza become the first and third line of the following stanzas; the first and third lines in the first stanza become the fourth and second lines in the last stanza. Some poets even rhyme the end words in an a-b-a-b pattern to add to the difficulty.

I attacked the pantoum form mathematically. Once I had my first line, I had my last. I wrote numbers down the left side of the page and just kept filling in lines as I had them. Getting to a logical end point of the poem was challenging. I literally cut apart the lines I wrote and kept rearranging them on my dining room table until I was satisfied. I actually found the process fun. It was reminiscent of the times before word processing. Students would cut apart the drafts of their term papers to rearrange paragraphs, then retype the whole thing! In 1982, white-out was considered high tech!

As I wrote more pantoums, I started to understand the form as a structure, a discipline. Foolishly, at the beginning of my writing career, I thought poetry would be easier to write than prose, as if one only had to write her thoughts, trailing them artfully down the page like e.e. cummings. Since poems were shorter, and seemingly "freestyle," I figured they had to be easier than writing prose, and certainly better than writing a scientific paper.

It didn't take me long to realize that shorter didn't equal easier. Shorter isn't easier in health care either. A patient's hospital stay is a lot shorter than it was twenty, ten, even five years ago. Now, the patient, nurse, and family have a lot to accomplish in a very short time, like a good poem.

"Coffee for One" was for an assignment in a writing class; otherwise, I doubt I would ever have tried this form. I started with a line from one of my unsuccessful poems: "Sometimes I sing to see if my voice works." I was single for many years before I met my husband. There were times the phone rang in the morning, and I would croak "Hello," voiceless because I hadn't spoken yet that day. I was trying to imagine what this would be like for someone who hadn't been alone before, such as a newly divorced man.

Imagination enters all good poems. To imagine is to conjure up something in our minds that is not in front of us at the moment. We might imagine something real in great detail, like a painting we saw at our last visit to the museum or how we felt on the first day of kindergarten. Imagination can also be a divergence from reality, the process of making up details, as in the previous poem—imagining that the newly divorced man would eat Pop-Tarts for breakfast; that he doesn't like to share the newspaper in the morning, and that he and his wife had fought about wet towels on the bed.

A typical admonition from writing instructors to new writers is "Show, Don't Tell." So instead of saying that a man is grieving for his wife, the writer writes that he doesn't change the sheets on his bed, or that he tucked her pillowcase into his briefcase.

Poems can come from anywhere our imagination takes us. We can place ourselves in the middle of an historical event. For example, what would it be like to be a soldier in Times Square, on V-J Day?

SAILOR EXPLAINS KISSING THE NURSE

After *V-J Day at Times Square, New York City, 1945*
PHOTOGRAPH BY ALFRED EISENSTAEDT

I didn't care who she was, this cloud of white
against a sea of gray pavement, littered with confetti
and crowds of seamen from Brooklyn Naval in
dress blues. Determined to kiss her

I swept her into my arms like a wave foaming
over the bow of a patrol boat. I hooked my arm around her
shoulders, and draped her so far backward,
one of her feet left dry land. How trusting

of her to dangle, as if over a cliff, and return the kiss
of a stranger amidst the revelers: office workers,
grandmothers, housewives, children all stopped to smile
as I covered her unsuspecting mouth, nestled

her cheek against my shoulder, tenaciously
as protecting a fresh pack of smokes from grabby
bunkmates. Her left arm slung back, her sleeve
a limp white flag of surrender.

The Pop! Pop! of a camera flash startled
us upright, she straightened her hem and needled
off through the crowd before the rewinding film
could even whir through the camera.

I think that Eisenstaedt's photograph has universal appeal. Almost everyone has seen it somewhere. I think I saw this photo long before I was a nurse, probably sitting on the couch with my father, leafing through *Time* books of photographs. The nurse's white uniform and cap held a lot of mystery for me. White was as universal a symbol of the nurse as the Red Cross or starched nursing cap. Not only did the white make it easy for this sailor to pick the nurse out of the crowd, the white angel is a symbol of caring. Nurses were held in high esteem during World War ii. No wonder the sailor wanted to kiss her in celebration!

In addition to imagination, this poem required a fair amount of research so that I could arrive at appropriate details. Books and the Internet were helpful, but the best part was interviewing my parents and my in-laws to hear what they remembered. The jubilation that came through their voices some fifty-five years after the event must have been a fraction of what they and all of America felt on V-J Day. My mother was in nyc that day and said, "There was paper everywhere. People just opened their windows and threw it out!" Photos such as this one keep emotion alive. I hoped to write a poem that would evoke emotion for a reader half a century later, and I wanted the poem to be credible even though I had not been born when this photograph was taken.

I've always wondered what the nurse was doing in the street at that moment. Was she just going to start her shift, or just leaving? Or did she step out of the hospital for a minute on her lunch break just to join the fun?

Over the years, several people claimed to be the soldier or the nurse. Eventually they were identified, but I like the idea of them being anonymous. Then, it could have been any nurse as the recipient of the happy and grateful smooch!

Probably everyone would agree that nurses, police, firefighters, and the military are in service positions. This photograph reminds me how artists serve society as well. Consider how the emotion stirred up by a photograph (or painting, sculpture, opera, poem) serves to enrich our world—for years.

At the $3 Car Wash

I know they look at my butt
as I wrestle the vacuum hose
between seats, under floor mats,
sucking up Cheerios and Goldfish
out of the Mom Mobile.
In and out of the car,
pitching juice boxes, shriveled fries,
I work up a sweat.

Just to check, I turn my head—
the guys in the matching windbreakers smile
and I narrow my eyes at them,
open the hatchback and crawl on all fours
to clean up dog hair imbedded
in grey carpet.

For less than a cup of cappuccino,
for less than five minutes,
these boys make me beautiful.
They know nothing of saddle bags,
stretch marks, or this deflated
pouch of skin I tuck into my jeans.

What can I do for you today, Gorgeous?
He tries to sell me the deluxe treatment:
whitewall wash, satin wax, bottom blast.
A hunk of soap in his hand, he scribbles
on my windshield, adds a smiley face,
punctuates the eyes.

Come on. Come on. He waves me towards him,
points right, left, raises a palm:
Neutral!
The surrender is best.
Water beats the sunroof, I dream
of a honeymoon waterfall in Tahiti.
Soapy tendrils shimmy on my hood,
down the sides of the van.
The rinse cycle steams the windows.
Heaters rise up and over me.

It's over too soon.
The conveyor thrusts me into sunlight,
dripping wet.
I look for a dirt road
on the way home.

This is my favorite poem because it was fun to write, it's fun to read to an audience, and I still smile every time I go through the car wash. At my three-dollar car wash, about halfway through the wash, is a flashing neon sign that says "Smile. This Is Fun."

Driving down Woodward Avenue, Detroit's thoroughfare for cruisers and folks just going from point A to point B, no guys check me out at the red lights anymore. Not too many guys flirt with a middle-aged gal in a van. But at the car wash on Woodward Avenue, I can count on just a smidgen of flirtation.

Soon after I sent this poem out, it was snatched up by a brand-new journal. When the poem finally was published, it was filled with typos. My heart sank. Typos are troublesome for the reader. As readers "hit" each mistake, they slow down. They have to decide what the misprinted word should have been. They have to guess and fill in words when editors leave them out. They start to doubt the poem. It truly interrupts the story and the music of the poem.

Perhaps this bothered me more than it would most poets due to my background as a nurse and a journalist. In each of these professions, errors are not tolerated. In newspapering, an error means, at the least, the dreaded "correction" in the next day's paper, or maybe a lawsuit, or even the loss of a job.

In nursing, an error could mean someone will die. In a profession with such high stakes, such dire consequences, I find I have low tolerance for errors. I have many dear friends who are leaders in their own professions: accountancy, retail, real estate, and even poetry. Sometimes they laugh about errors they've made on the job. When they complain about not getting the sale, the promotion, the grant, I have to bite my lip. I want to say, "Get over it. No one died."

It will be a delight to see this poem reprinted correctly and to finally be proud to pass the book around. Maybe I'll show the car wash guys.

ARMY NURSES, VIETNAM, 1966

After the Vietnam Women's Memorial, Washington, D.C.
GLENNA GOODACRE, *Sculptor*

Too exhausted to swat the flies
that buzz their hair, three nurses
sit back-to-back on sandbags
to rest, to wait for the wounded
soldier to be choppered out, handed
over to the USS Sanctuary floating off Vietnam.

Among the bamboo trees of Phu Nhon, Vietnam,
one of the nurses holds the flyer,
stretches her arm, reaches her hand
across his chest: a pieta of nurse
and soldier, her limbs wound
around him to contain this awkward package

slipping from her grasp. She opens her bag,
wets her bandanna to shield him from Vietnam
sun, cools his forehead, covers his wounded
eyes until a surgeon can attempt repairs, mid-flight.
There is too much damage, but still she nurses,
grieving the loss of yet another handsome

face. To keep him on her lap, she grasps a handful
of the soldier's shirt. A plastic bag
rustles in his pocket. The nurse
peeks at the photo he carries in this Vietnam
jungle: a young woman with flowing hair. *Fly
High, Love you,* she wrote with curlicues winding

into hearts. Placing the photo in its flimsy bag,
the nurse seals it, tucks it back, wounded.
The faces of all the Joes, Bobs, Gerrys and Smittys fly
through her mind, blur with the rows of body bags
that carried them from Vietnam—
last words spoken, spoken to their nurse.

Lifting her chin, rising to full height, the second nurse
turns black eyes to the sky. Hot wind
stirs the tight curls underneath her cap. In Vietnam,
unarmed, she reaches back to lay a hand
on her comrade's elbow, touching her baggy
sleeve, waiting for rescue, to fly

out. The third nurse kneels, motionless as a butterfly
regaining strength after tearing from its silk cocoon.
The fine red dust of Vietnam coats her helmet, her hands.

In 1966 I was in the fifth grade. Daily, we prayed for peace; we prayed for the
soldiers in Vietnam. I don't remember praying for any women over there, and
I wasn't really aware that women served in battle zones until M*A*S*H on TV.

This was the most technically difficult poem I have ever written. The form
of this poem is a sestina, a form requiring that the same words (or variation of
those words: hand, handful, handsome) end the six-line stanzas in a prescribed
order. The last stanza (three lines, or a tercet, also called an *envoi*) uses two of
the end words in each line.

The week before I wrote this poem, I visited the Vietnam Women's Memorial. It was 2000, on Memorial Day. I was visiting my sister, who lived in the D.C. area, and when she asked, "What do you want to do this trip?" I mentioned the memorial.

At the memorial that day, there were nurse and non-nurse veterans present to honor their fallen comrades. Some sang, some read poems or letters or spoke of their memories. All of the mementos left at the memorial were moving: a doctor had shaped six wreaths out of barbed wire for six nurses who had died; there were flags tucked all over the sculpture, a rose placed in a "nurse's" bronzed hand, and notes left in Ziploc bags at the bronze nurses' booted feet. After this experience, not to write a poem would have been to abandon the nurses.

When I was in graduate school for my MSN, nursing students and RNs all over the country were raising money for this memorial. I remember contributing ten dollars, which in 1980 was a lot of money for me. Once the memorial was paid for (by nurses!) the government did not want this memorial anywhere near "The Wall." I was incredulous. It was the first time I realized how little status women and nurses had.

So nurses started writing letters. Lots of letters. They testified before congress. They made phone calls. Finally, on November 11, 1993, the dedication ceremony took place. I was disappointed that I could not be there for the dedication; however, one of the nurse executives from my hospital was there, front and center. It was a day for all nurses.

The end words on each line are very important to the sestina. Finally, I wised up and carefully chose end words that could be varied in many ways, thus offering a variety of meanings that would help propel the story along. Sestinas generally do have a story, making the poems a narrative as well. This poem was exhausting. It took me a week of continuous effort and brought me to a difficult realization. At the time I wrote it, I was considering going back to graduate school for an MFA in poetry. This poem knocked the wind out of me: I was crabby, the housekeeping didn't get done, the dog didn't get walked, AND forget home-cooked meals! The family suffered. I realized nope, it's not time for me to go back to school. I suppose this was better than having already enrolled in a program and paid a semester's tuition! Now I am much more empathetic when a young person says "it's not the time" to go to nursing school to get her BSN or her specialty certification.

This poem was accepted for a nursing anthology. The wise editor suggested some edits to streamline the poem. At first I freaked, because with some of the changes, the poem was no longer a "by the book" sestina. I couldn't deny that the editor's changes made the poem less clunky. She varied from the rule book for the benefit of the poem. I emailed the editor and told her that I liked her changes but was mourning the loss of the form. She went over the poem again and added some of the end words back.

How many times do nurses need to break the rules for the benefit of the patient? How many of us have not bent rules for our patients? When my father was in a university hospital, two weeks before his death from leukemia, the nurses let Dad (diabetic) have ice cream with his birthday cake. They just increased the next dose of his insulin. When Dad told his nurse that he just drank a smuggled-in "Perfect Canadian Manhattan with a twist," his nurse smiled and said, "Just one?"

Part of life as a nurse is knowing which rules to break and when. This is also true for the poet. Part of the life of a nurse is also knowing when to accept help. My gut reaction when I saw how the editor improved my sestina was to feel embarrassed that I couldn't do that myself. She had made it a better poem. Hundreds of times, my patients got better care because I had the consultation and help of another nurse.

I have a favorite line in this poem, which I think is the crux of the nurse-patient relationship in this memorial sculpture: "last words spoken, spoken to their nurse." I don't think I have ever felt such intense intimacy with anyone as the moment of holding the dying patient in the absence of his or her family. As a young nurse, I was overwhelmed with the burden of being the last person to witness a breath or hear a last message; I felt tremendously guilty in passing it along and felt, "if only I could have kept the patient alive another fifteen minutes for the family" to hear it themselves. Did the family fault me? Now I know that some patients wait for their families to leave so they can die without burdening them.

I learned early not to promise a patient that he or she wouldn't die. I cared for a patient who was three weeks postpartum on a medical unit. She was anxious, couldn't breathe, and the CPR team was on the way. She kept saying, "I'm going to die." I said, "No you're not." She died. One truth about nursing is that you don't ever know what will happen next. I can't imagine what it was like for these Vietnam nurses to see the "mass cals" (mass casualties) come through the "doors" of their medevac units. Young men, covered in mud, their own guts. When the young wounded said, "I'm going to die," I'm sure those nurses were wiser than I was.

I entered nursing school for two reasons. I knew I liked helping people, and I wanted to have job security. I had been a "volunteer" during my high school years. I worked in the hospital flower room, unwrapping flowers, then delivering flowers and newspapers to patients' rooms. I would look at the nurses in their white caps and white uniforms and think they were angels. I became comfortable with the hospital environment and knew that I could fit in. As a "senior project" at Marian High School, I worked as a volunteer in a hemodialysis unit. The staff nurses there treated me very kindly. I was touched by the stories of the patients and impressed by how important nurses were to their overall well-being.

Although I was torn between studying English or nursing, my father felt strongly that I needed to have a career in which I could have great job security. "You'll always have a job as a nurse." He felt strongly that I should get a BSN. "A degree is your ticket," he said, "to all kinds of opportunities in life."

I must confess that I was terrified of taking chemistry in college and afraid to major in nursing because of it. Luckily, my college was a small school with a terrific faculty-to-student ratio. The professor who taught freshman chemistry went out of her way to help the nursing students succeed, by extending office hours, extra tutoring, etc.

I view my *writing self* as a poet, but it wasn't always that way. I started out writing short fiction and won several awards for short stories in high school. Many years later I had one short story published in *The MacGuffin*. It was a "life into fiction" story that came from my memories of a patient. During the first twenty years after nursing school, I concentrated on writing scholarly papers for nursing journals and published about fifty. I earned a journalism degree then wrote health-related articles for the popular press. My expertise in journalism helped me to obtain the position of associate editor at *Plastic Surgical Nursing*. At about the same time I became the internal communications coordinator (responsible for the employee newspaper, video news program, management news, etc.) at a one thousand-bed bed hospital. I worked in that position for three years but had to return to the patient bedside. I really missed caring for patients and knowing at the end of every day that I made some kind of difference in someone's life.

I think of myself as a poet, but that is a fairly recent thing. What are the credentials for a poet? Perhaps an MFA. But there are plenty of famous poets before us without any formal training. I began writing poetry at the age of sixteen, before nursing school. In nursing, it is clear that when a person receives an RN license, he or she can say, "I am a registered nurse." Even though I don't have an official credential as a poet, I can comfortably say that I am a writer of poetry, now that I have a shelf full of magazines in which I am published.

Of the books I read as a child, my favorite was *The Velveteen Rabbit*. I read all of the *Nancy Drew* books under my bed covers with a flashlight. Maybe it's peculiar, but I never read any of the *Cherry Ames* books or other "nurse" books.

I recall my first poem in 1972; I was trying to imitate e.e. cummings. I am sure the poem was awful. I wrote another poem in high school, which I have since lost, that sticks out in my mind. In the high school yearbook, each senior could list her accomplishments or write a quote after her name in the senior directory. One girl, who I did not know well, used two lines from a poem I wrote. I didn't know whether to be embarrassed or proud. She did not credit me, and at the time I was relieved. It was the first time I realized that my words could mean anything to anyone.

Many times I've taken an extended break from writing, for example, after a big exhausting project or a big disappointment (rejection). Then, something happens in my life that I want to hang on to: a moment with my daughter, a work of art, an "aha" moment when I understand something in a different way. So I write it down. At least in poetry, what we write belongs to us. We can always keep a copy of the words. I have an Aunt, eighty-plus years, who is a wonderful artist. When she sells a painting, she is pleased, but her heart breaks because she has to see it go, usually to far-flung places where she will never see it again. She keeps photographs of her works, but I don't think it's the same. Poets are lucky that we never lose what we write.

I have a lot of journals to write in but don't carry any of them with me. I keep one in my car, one by the bed, several in my office, and one *might* be in my purse. New poems are often started on paper napkins or the back of an envelope. I often work on poems while I am in the pickup line, waiting for my daughter at school. One started in the checkout line at the grocery store. One of my teachers told me to always keep an index card in my jeans pocket. Every time she e-mails me or sends a card, she writes "still keeping those index cards in your pocket?" I'd hate to tell her that most of my clothes don't have pockets.

If I do sit down with the purpose of writing poetry, I first sharpen a dozen pencils. I like the smell. I usually write on deadline. Students in journalism school learn to write on deadline. In News Writing 101, the teacher would give us the facts (in a scrambled order) then set the timer and we would have to write the news story. Fast. Accurate. No Mistakes. A lot like nursing. It reminds me of that end-of-shift frenzy when the nurse charts what she should have been writing all day, but there wasn't time!

In journalism school, my teachers and classmates would tell me I was good at noticing and then reporting on details in a story. I have heard the same about the details in my poems. I have to give the credit to one of my instructors in nursing school, and I am ashamed I can't remember which one it was. My college had a small but beautiful campus. The nursing professor told us that in order to sharpen our observational skills, we should try to notice something different on the way to class each day. Even if we took the same route from the dorm room to the nursing building, there would be something different to notice: freshly trimmed shrubs, chalk marks on the sidewalk, a new face. It has become a life-long habit, and now I play this "game" with my daughter on our drive to school in the morning. She's better at it than I am now, but of course, I'm watching the road.

It is the nature of nursing that we have good observational skills. We call it assessment, the first step in the nursing process. Nurses also learn good interviewing skills. This helped me immensely in journalism school too.

Nursing has offered me a number of interesting jobs over the years: staff nursing in a variety of areas, home care, teaching, advance practice nursing, and administration, not to mention that flexible schedules have allowed me to pursue other interests, have a family, work at school, write, sew quilts—it goes on and on. I have no regrets that I became a nurse.

Nursing feeds my life as a poet. After spending all day caring for others, I have to write some of it down in order to care for myself. Sometimes I write the events of the day in a journal, then close it and never look at it again. Some things are too painful to revisit or they just aren't that important.

Sometimes there are days that are so memorable in their rewards or horrors that I write nothing down at the end of the day. Often, these are the days that haunt me and emerge in poems or stories a decade later. When it comes to writing the poem about the patient, it is my recall, filtered through my imagination and empathy, that I use, not notes.

My patients trust me with their care, their pain, their vulnerabilities, their stories. They teach me about myself, and offer me an appreciation of the world that I wouldn't have on my own.

POETRY PUBLICATIONS

Spencer's poetry publications include the following book:

Waiting for Ice to Melt. Chapbook. Self-published, 2003.

Spencer has poems published in the following journals:

American Poetry Monthly; Bark; Bonfire Review; California Quarterly; Chimes; Clackamas Review; Driftwood Review; Ekphrasis; FAN; Inkwell; LUNGFULL; MacGuffin; Mediphors; Off the Coast; 100 Words; Potpourri; Red Cedar Review; Red Rock Review; Rosebud; Terminus; U.S. Catholic; Welcome Home.

Spencer's poetry is included in the following anthologies:

Intensive Care: More Poetry and Prose by Nurses. Ed. Cortney Davis and Judy
    Schaefer. Iowa City: Univ. of Iowa Press, 2003.
Only a River between Us. Ed. Kathleen Ripley Leo. Detroit, Mich.: Detroit
    Women Writers, 2001.
The Space Between. Ed. Mary Ann Wehler. Troy, Mich.: Classroom and Com-
    munity Publishing, 2001.
A Time to Speak. Ed. Mary Ann Wehler, Mary Jo Firth Gillett, and M. L. Liebler.
    Troy, Mich.: Classroom and Community Publishing, 2000.

Constance Studer

෯෧

Nurses, like their patients, are often caught in the grip of suffering. Like some of the other nurses in this book, Studer writes about her own illness, attributed to a vaccine, something we expect to protect us. In the following pages, she articulates her trek, guided by the new maps of literary devices and exquisite observation. She holds nothing back. Maps become veins and arteries and healing rivers; words become salvation. She writes curiously of fellow nurses who perceived her as less serious once they learned of her writing workshops and graduate classes. She perseveres, her lives merging into a new creative being. She learns to "layer metaphors and emotions" so that she can take it all in. The ultimate destination is a place of joy rather than despair when she writes, "I have no answers, only two hands."

DEAR DR. WILLIAMS, DEAR POET

It's all about pace
planting palms within loamy skin
excavating stories buried deep within bone, you whisper

as I bob on the rim of the university bubble,
float past preachers and salesmen certain
they have the antidote to disease and famine.

Poem. Steady eye at the hurricane center
of flu epidemics and cancer clusters,
supplication to spare a son, a father.

Hours stolen between patients,
scribbling poems on the back of envelopes,
furtive game of test and balance.

Lay cold metal ear against shivering flesh,
listen to the swish of deficient valves
as the anxious heart gallops across open meadow.

My offering is about Carla who bled,
whom I've just left alone inside all those tubes
and wires that need tending,

an innocent who didn't know that the miracle
keeping her heart dancing—*pacemaker*—could also be dangerous,
the reason I arrived cold, wet, late.

Pens carry steady light down into the body's labyrinth,
part and weave incisions bloom with looped handles,
grey roses, white gardenias. Into the netherworld

grasp red muscle, yellow fat between metal teeth,
part and weave. Your voice in my ear: *Never mind*
the phone, that mad thing, that curse,

words demand to be born
between calming a man bronzed by leukemia,
child pregnant with child.

House still, my son warm in his bed,
words blow through leaves calling.
What medicine takes apart,

poetry breathes in whole. Knife and pen join hands,
take up the dance,
whirl and glide and spin face-to-face,

arms encircling arms as they debride scar tissue,
excise pendulous tumors,
sing lyrical songs *a capella*

with bell-like harmony of hemostats and knives,
wounds healed by a tiny thread of ink.
Next shift Carla's cheeks are bright peonies

and my poem—dancing its wild flamenco
within her chest—has just earned
the only prize it will ever need.

VOICES IN THE BOOKS LINING my shelves call to me. I pick up Emerson and his words sing, *The poet is the only true doctor.* Freud whispers, *Everywhere I go I find a poet has been there before me.* Flaubert croons, *One does not choose one's subject matter, one submits to it.* And from the twentieth-century doctor-poet William Carlos Williams, who scribbled poems in scattered moments between delivering babies and shooting antibiotics into the buttocks of scream-ing children: *It is difficult / to get the news from poems / yet men die miserably every day / for lack / of what is found there.*

The first time I saw a caduceus it was hanging on the wall of my stepfather's office. Back in the late 1950s, Dr. Kenneth Browne was a general practitioner in a small farming community in northern Ohio. The caduceus, that most revered holy symbol, the scepter and two serpents, the emblem of life associ-ated with physical and spiritual health. My bedroom was at the top of the stairs of our home; I often heard odd bits of conversation as it floated up from Dad Browne's office. *Need to cut out this mole. Is it cancer, Doctor? Won't know until I do the biopsy. Wait and see.* The summer before I entered nurse's training, he sometimes let me help.

I watched as he listened with the stethoscope for wheezes or bubbles or rales. He tapped with his middle finger as he listened for an echo, a timbre that would tell whether fluid or a mass was lodged between the lung and his hand. It was from him that I learned that hands and heart can speak more clearly than words.

Nursing is monitors chugging and paying close attention to the body. Nursing is sudden death and standing at the head of the bed, bagging and saying, *You'll be okay, Mr. Bennett. You'll feel us pressing on your chest.* All he'll remember later are lights and tunnels. Coronary care is high tech and chest pain and fear of bypass open-heart surgery and calling the attendant at mid-night. Coronary care is lidocaine and sodium bicarbonate and three hundred watts of electric shock to the heart. *Does the patient have a pulse? Give the epi now.* Nursing is a fight for the right to provide nursing care; it is a circle of fatigue around the eyes. Nurses are the unhappy spouses in this marriage to medicine. The marriage isn't working, but no one knows how to fix it. Patients are the latchkey children of this volatile union, the innocents who experience the inadequacy of the health-care safety net.

Just say the words *intensive care nurse* and images can swirl out of focus: smashed skulls, stapled backs, shaved heads, curved incisions, bandage turbans, surgical drains, crani caps. I've stood in the hall and felt the air being sucked out of the room as a surgeon left after telling a young wife that her husband had an inoperable brain tumor. I've witnessed burned skin turn pink, pain numbed, eyesight saved, walking restored. Our patients arrived with hope: ranchers from the Western Slope, a teacher from Pueblo, a butcher from Telluride, a CEO from a software firm, a homeless man. We were the ones who eased them out of their jean jackets and blazers and three-piece suits, tied up the back of their flimsy gowns.

The heart, that complicated mixture of dependency and splendid independence. To be able to listen to the human heart, to draw meaning from its slightest vibrations or whispers, to take a droplet of blood and perceive its vital balances, to convert electric markings into precise knowledge are only science to doctors. But to the patient they are powers that come from the gods.

I was working full time in Intensive Care–Coronary Care when I was accepted in the Masters of Arts Program in Creative Writing at the University of Colorado. Every week at the poetry workshop, I was aware of how different my world was from that of my fellow students. Not only was I older than the other students, I was also working full time and a single parent of a young son. As I listened to students arguing about the length of a term paper, my mind was still with the family of a person we'd just saved in the unit. I was in the workshop to learn the craft of poetry, to be around other people who loved literature, to get my work critiqued, to make sense of all those images of pain and human idiosyncrasies and battling egos.

When my fellow nurses found out that I was taking writing workshops and graduate classes, a curious thing happened. Suddenly I was perceived as not being as serious about nursing as I'd been before. The thought of changing careers was the furthest thing from my mind. Since no one asked what writing meant to me, I never told them that writing is a way of life as well as a vocation, a process, a journey, more than a destination. Writing becomes a life-sustaining habit, like exercise or eating three meals a day. I wanted to tell my fellow nurses that writing and nursing go together like a long, peaceful marriage where each partner takes turns crying and consoling, arguing and reconciling. The marriage lasts because both partners know they've been heard, understood, and accepted in spite of all their imperfections.

I write to create an alternative universe where I can pretend that oceans are pristine, where hospitals are no longer needed. Writing is a mingling of sweet and sour, yin and yang, terror and tingle. A legal high when a sentence works or a poem tells me what it wants to say. Writing, that trancelike state where distractions disappear, anxiety is put on hold; a feeling of flow, endorphins, natural opiates; that room where I can close the door and be safe and whole.

In life, like in writing a poem, one of the most difficult lessons is learning how to layer pain in metaphors and emotions so that you can take it in. Layer it like the stroke of fingers on an arm, like the stanzas in a psalm.

Writing is like nursing in many ways. You never feel as though what you have to offer is good enough. You're never done. You have to pay close attention to details or it will die. You have to keep the faith, persevere, see it through. People are the primary ingredient in both. You must be willing to reassess at a moment's notice and embark on another course. Sometimes radical surgery is needed in order for it to heal. Telling a story, listening to another person's, is what sacred means.

Hawk, Winter

Bedtime prayers move apartment walls
giving life to silence as if wings were rising
outside the window.

Snug under his quilt, I read my son his favorite book,
Where the Sidewalk Ends, as snow presses hard against the sill.
Somewhere there is always war,

a desert or city ghetto where boys try to defeat
the enemy with stones,
innocent bodies stacked like cordwood.

Life, that white chip that can disappear as quickly
as a roll of dice while the soul goes on.
Overnight the pond behind our building

is one frozen blank eye. Overnight trees have bared naked arms.
Out of nowhere a hawk dives,
its eye a great reticulated yellow orb.

I pull my son into my arms just in time,
my child who will always be too young to wade
through sauna jungles,

to hide waist deep in mined rice paddies,
to sleep with one eye open.
Late evening sun transforms the prism in our window

into a rainbow on the wall
all the colors within the body: *golden fat, soft*
and pulpy like the inside of an orange,

pink intestines, crimson pools that fade to purple.
Our president comes on TV delivering the rat-a-tat-tat
of big guns. *Friendly fire. Collateral damage.*

I turn down the volume and watch stern men move silent mouths
but still hear their slogans: *God is in our cockpit.*
I am stronger than you are. Thumb in nose. Far away smart bombs

hone in on targets that have eyes
and hearts, shades of red bleed into the desert.
My hands steady the dulcimer

while my son's small fingers caress the strings,
bestow tiny bursts of heavenly sharps
and flats, his touch

the trembling wingtip of a dove.
Light candles for his seventh birthday,
angel food cake, a magician's set with black cape

and gold wand. Balloons filled with ghosts that drift toward heaven
if I let go for a second. My love blows soapy bubbles through a ring
that gleams with his brightest breath.

Gentle puffs float through winter dusk along the rim
of the window sill, out into the suddenly warm night.
May the wings I heard be angels

instead of hawks. May the magician's wand
make war vanish. May our world not end with a headline,
a slogan, a fiction redder than the Cedars of Lebanon:

Pax Americana.
Fang baring.
Brilliant display of plumage.

There is an African saying, "When two elephants fight, it's the grass that suffers most." *If I just find the perfect words, people will wake up. Our planet is in danger. Our obsession with big cars is changing our climate. We can't take the chance of waging another war. Forests denuded. Wolves shot. Eagles poisoned.* "Hawk, Winter," written during the Gulf War conflict in 1991, is about the fear that lies beneath skin, beneath the surface of a pond, fear deep within my heart about the future that my generation will leave for our children. In 2003 we are headed for yet another war.

The medicine I learned as a nurse was full of military metaphors: *Attack, mission, defense.* Disease is the foreign country. Search and Destroy is the battle cry. Body as battleground. *Bring in the heavy arsenal of drugs and surgery. Fire shots of warning.* Nursing is as front line as medicine gets. Nursing requires a computer brain and a wrestler's muscles and the heart of a lover. Nurses are marathon runners who never reach the finish line, never win a trophy. Nursing is paying attention to the little things: Knowing which vein to try. Knowing that Mr. Lane prefers to lie on his left side with a pillow behind his back and between his legs since that decreases pain in his lower spine. Hospitals are year-long Halloweens, with their tricks or treats, their masks of fear and laughter.

In 1984 I was forced to retire from nursing due to total physical disability. Four years later, after many biopsies, hospitalizations, and consultations with specialists, my doctors concurred that my illness—systemic vasculitis, systemic lupus, glomerulonephritis—was caused by the Heptavax-B vaccine I'd received while working as a nurse. I always thought I was a compassionate nurse, but until I lay in a hospital bed myself, was given the wrong medication, was treated badly by an arrogant doctor, I had no idea what patients went through.

In between doctor appointments and hospitalizations and raising my son, I spent sleepless nights trying to define pain. Maybe if I could put it into words, it would be more manageable. Pain was still lying awake, alone, at 2 A.M. in a hospital room as needles dissected my feet, legs, hands, abdomen. Pain was the mountain I climbed every day in order to have lunch with a friend or enjoy a movie. Being a patient was being palpated and drummed and poked with needles. Being a patient meant being awakened at four for blood pressure checks and hanging modesty in the closet along with my jeans and sweater. Being a patient meant doctors and nurses and kitchen workers parading through my room on their schedules instead of mine. Being a patient was a free fall through space and time, the shock of impermanence.

Try this natural healer, my neighbor said. My friend Barbara gave me crystals—*amethyst, carnelian, coral, lapis, obsidian, tourmaline*—to carry around in a little brown bag. I tried them all: faith healing, meditation, crystals, therapeutic pool, megavitamins, Cytoxan, prednisone, vasodilators, plasmapheresis, prayer. Twice a day I stood in front of my bedroom mirror and told myself, *Your body is healing. The pain is gone. Your veins and arteries are rivers, circling round, running back freely toward your heart. Hold positive thoughts and images that instill peace.*

Nineteen years later, I know that, although I may not be able to heal my body, I can heal my life: Spending the morning writing. Sitting on the shore of Grand Lake, watching ducks float by as hawks do their call-and-response act high up in the trees. Sinking down into a warm tub. Laughing with good friends over life's latest absurdity. Making a positive contribution whenever I can. Raising my son and being a friend, a sister, a writer.

Body language is a foreign language slowly translated, often painfully understood. Just to dance, to be, arms up, legs stretching out. Constantly testing, teasing the boundaries, with a turn of the head, a touch. Breath follows breath. Nothing else matters.

HIGHER LEARNING

Our unit becalmed,
responsibility almost over,
an admission arrives
    domestic abuse
    we know this woman well,
    the ER nurse says.
We couple the fragile woman
to bubbling tubes and catheters
and monitors unconscious,
fine skin with deeply incised
cuts by both eyes,

heart tattooed on her thigh.
Nurse eyes and brain register
    closed head injury,
    pupils react sluggishly to light,
    compound fracture right arm,
while my heart grieves how her brain
has backslidden down skull,
how glaze seals eyes she can't open,
legs stiff as aluminum,
hands closing over nothing,
our hands the same size

on the steering wheel
driving west that hot July night on the highway
not knowing how far the desert stretches,
miles hold the power to heal,
speed the analgesia,
love my son asleep in the back seat.

Sue did nothing but fall asleep
in her bed and will wake up
in ICU *maybe not* tubes bubble
as I tally up numbers

truck drivers honk as I put my fist
of bright lights in their eyes

machines breathe hope
plastic tubes nourish

through all those one-stoplight towns
and six-lane cities,
one more woman traveling west

computers translate
every tick into language only God
can decipher. It's not enough
to know how cell bodies
and sharp tentacles touch enabling speech

praying in the Last Chance Motel
a temporary home with a lock on the door
and a bed that holds us both

to know how electrical impulses
jump from nerve to muscle
pulsing blood down
ever smaller highways,
not enough to memorize the names of muscles
and arteries of that four-chambered organ
the size of a fist prone to attack and to failure
why love turns into attack
and counterattack

Lord let me learn help me
find nouns adjectives,
let us see sun rise over mountains

and I have no answers,
only two hands
rubbing lotion into my sister's skin.

The map that I followed to Boulder was a long, tortuous one extending from Ohio, where I was born and raised, to Amsterdam, where my husband was a student, to Illinois, back to Amsterdam, to Ithaca, New York (where my husband was again a student), and finally to Colorado. In 1973, Boulder was a small university town of twenty thousand souls snuggled up against the Rocky Mountains. Boulder, with its semi-arid foothills and Martian-like sunsets, is a solid middle-American community replete with fitness fanatics and liberal environmentalists and Buddhists, with more than its share of Ph.D.s waiting tables. Family is the first map of the world.

July 1973. We were four for the road: my sister Pat, my niece Diane, my baby son Christopher, and me. It began to rain. When I turned on the wind-shield wipers, I heard them whisper *Heartsick* one way and *Wanderlust* the other, back and forth. Rain fell on cars as they moved slowly ahead, behind, alongside. I drove, tense against the noise of the car, the air conditioner, the noise of unfamiliarity. My son's whimpers turned into sobs. Pat leaned over and pulled my baby from his car seat. Wet diaper. Hunger. The sharp smell of baby poop filled the air. The usual basic miseries were in my son's wail. *Does he know? Is he missing his father already?*

Ten years of marriage had split my skin. At the last moment I called Pat and asked her if she'd like to go on a trip. *Where are you going?* she asked. *Boulder, Colorado,* I whispered, as if saying the words would make it real. I couldn't explain to my sister that my marriage was over. That I had to leave. It was the same feeling I'd had when I'd been driving with Chris in the foothills around Ithaca and had thought I was following the map, only the road kept getting narrower, changing from asphalt to dirt. I was nervous because there was a cliff on the left and a drop-off on the right and I could not see to the bottom. No way to turn around. I'd always thought love was a two-way street instead of a dirt road leading nowhere.

Life can change in one minute. I was working as evening supervisor at the local hospital when I received the Heptavax-B vaccine. August 1983. Summer heat was receding into one of the most beautiful Colorado autumns I could remember. Aspens had their brightness knobs turned up to their highest levels: stained-glass reds, crackling oranges, browns side by side like mosaic tiles. Colors jumped out in stark relief against a cloudless blue canvas. Rashes appeared, fever, hypertension. All I wanted to do was sleep. My parenting skills settled uneasily into automatic pilot, my twelve-year-old son on cruise control, holding course, steady, the brightest spot on my horizon. October 28, 1983. After a night of intense pain and fever, I called in sick, pulled sheets up over my shaking body. The shift the evening before was the last one I would ever work as a nurse.

I replayed this scenario at least twenty times in the next two years: I sat in a doctor's office nervously waiting for him to probe various parts of my body and history that were not usually open to public scrutiny. My worry filled the room, air heavy with awareness that decisions were being made that would change my future. The doctor knew my age, weight, blood pressure, medications, past and present symptoms. I agreed to this, stripped myself of reticence, along with my slacks and sweater, and answered his questions as part of an implicit agreement: *patient tells all; doctor cures all.* Tomorrow was always the day the doctors would have the answers. I was thrown into a game of diagnostic roulette: *Isolate the symptom. Pinpoint its source. Devise a compensation mechanism for all the life changes.* I was treated with prednisone, anti-malarial drugs, Cytoxin, and almost two years of immunmodulatory therapy which included plasmapheresis.

The twentieth-century German poet Rainer Maria Rilke's answer to uncertainty was, "Have patience with everything that remains unsolved in your heart. Try to love the *questions themselves* like locked rooms and like books that are written in a very foreign language. Do not look for the answers. They cannot be given you because you could not live them. It is a question of experiencing everything. At present you need to *live* the question. Perhaps you will gradually, without even noticing it, find yourself experiencing the answer some distant day" (*Letters to a Young Poet, Classic Wisdom Collection,* Translated by Joan M. Burnham, San Rafael, Calif.: New World Library, 1992, p. 35).

Make an intuitive leap and the logic comes later. There's a whole other reality that can't be reached by intellect, or by following a road map, or by linear thinking. When a person is ill, bodily events are magnified. A new map of the body is drawn, with detours around the sites that no longer function as before. Body and mind are no longer separate. Mind united with flesh. Pieces of the great puzzle scatter and reassemble under my feet as I research vaccine-related illnesses at Denison Library, affiliated with the University of Colorado Health Sciences Center in Denver. Days in the library become fluid, mornings blending seamlessly into evenings. *I think your illness was caused by the Heptavax-B vaccine,* my immunologist says to me in October 1986, but it's two more years before he puts it in writing. I want someone to knock on my door and say, *We're sorry.* But that would admit wrongdoing and that will never happen. New drugs are not tested on women before they appear in the marketplace. Pharmaceutical companies have always taken men's bodies as the norm. We women are too complicated, with all our hormones and ovaries and breasts.

Nine months after submitting a Freedom of Information request about adverse events related to the Heptavax-B vaccine, I receive a large carton containing a computer printout from the Vaccine Adverse Event Reporting

System. I note with a sinking heart all the vascular problems recorded: heart attack, stroke, perforated bowel, as well as milder symptoms such as rashes, muscular pain, fever:

> *Number 333383: A fifty-eight-year-old male physician who developed myalgias, arthralgias, fatigue, serous otititis media, transient loss of vision in one eye and multiple peripheral neuropathies following the third injection of Heptavax-B...* *He is currently being treated with Cytoxan and prednisone for a polyarteritis-like illness.* (VAERS, Vaccine Adverse Event Reporting System, computer printout, Atlanta, GA: Center for Disease Control, 1986).

Prayer needs no map, no instruction manual. Pain begins when I open my eyes, sip my coffee. Medications are as essential as food. Bed is my second home. The world outside gets dressed in suits and trips off to office or classroom. I no longer fit into this world of corporate ladders and performance evaluations and net worth. It's up to me to create my day, prioritize my life. No one will return and save me.

I drive up Fourmile Canyon, sit by a mountain stream as it sings through a huddle of Aspen. This canyon, with its pictographs and petroglyphs, is alive with spirits. I feel another presence, as if someone were pushing me from behind. A sense of coming through, seeing beyond. Cirrus clouds feather the sky, eternal eyes watching. Translucent leaves, backlit by the sun, glimmer like gold dust. I close my eyes, sit and wait. Peace. Harmony. Silence. *Now what?* I ask the clouds. Out of the silence comes an answer: *What is needed is here and will always come.* And it does. *Listen to the deep source of wisdom within yourself. Tell the truth. Keep asking, is this true for me? Have courage to follow where the questions lead.*

ROSE

> *She was fine an hour ago* her parents say
> and I believe them,
> their tiny girl snuggled in a yellow jumpsuit covered with daisies,
> plump baby arms, lips a scarlet thread.
> *Her name is Rose,* the mother says. I write down the facts:
>
> *well baby born full term,*
> *not eating the past day, three hours*
> *of significant fever, irritability,* all the while worried.
> It's just the look of her, an intuition
> that warns me. Curls cluster like black grapes,

her cheeks a bouquet fresh from the garden. Her weak cry
the singing of a robin just broken from its shell. Pale skin veiled in purple dots.
We puncture the ivory of her arms with needles, *barely speak,*
work fast. She whimpers and then doesn't resist.
In spite of everything we do, she pools,

coalesces, darkens as purple spreads
across her belly. Fixes her blue eyes on mine.
The eyes of a fawn by the river, waiting to drink.
Mother stands, lips parted, staring, a pillar of salt.
Father covers his face. There is no one to go to them.

Force a tube down her mouth,
her teeth a flock of sheep, *tilt back*
her silken head, pump her mottled chest,
push penicillin, breathe for her,
preserve blood in tubes, *no time to think, hold the tiny*

intravenous in one hand, stroke her hair with the other,
my love, my little sister.
The electrocardiogram alarms
running her story too fast. Baby eyes
roll up into long lashes. *Where has she gone?*

Back to the first garden,
the bed of spices,
the garland of roses just opening.   The line is flat,
has been for some time,
but we cannot believe, refuse to stop.

When I try to tell the parents,
my tongue is granite. She has set a seal on our hearts.
Branded us. *Pull the curtain but I cannot wrap her tiny body*
in coarse white sheets. Run, lovely little one,
run and be a young deer on the mountain.

Every hospital wears a mask of polished floors and papered feet, gleaming
machinery. Scalpels part skin. The sharp, clean smell of measured emotions.
Here masks are pulled off: a child with a broken arm, a mother with a suckling
child. Shock trails in behind an accident victim, the numbing ache of those
with loved ones who now lie still and breathless in windowless rooms.

"Rose" is one of several poems that I've written about taking care of criti-cally ill children. Often, names are gone but faces remain. *How to put grief into words? Tomorrow I'll be a better writer. A better nurse.* It never gets easier for either profession. Parents turn to statues before my eyes. Then there's our grief, all of us working so hard to save her life. Grief that mustn't be displayed, must be postponed in order to deal with the crisis at hand. Writing this poem was an expiation of guilt as well as grief. I couldn't save this little girl, so I wanted to keep her alive in words.

I write to bear witness. Because I must. Because of my love affair with a blank notebook and pen. The abstract painting of black ink on white paper turns into the image of a clear lake that I can sit beside and be at peace. Writ-ing is thought of as cerebral work while nursing is more physical (although cerebral as well), but trying to divide body and mind is ludicrous. The breath that starts a poem is the same breath used to resuscitate a patient. Both start in the body and enliven the mind. Both see through to the heart of things. Both nursing and writing are getting down on your hands and knees, getting dirty, inspecting life at close range. Language comes in pumping rhythms, like prayer or song. Like blood pumping through the heart. The writer's struggle is against the demon of that which resists being put into words. To surrender to the love-hate, happiness-misfortune dichotomy called literature. To follow the dark path from intuition to understanding. An exercise in freedom.

Hands of a nurse give backrubs, hands of a writer hold a pen. Both have known rejection and bear pale lines of old scars. My hands have diapered my baby son and made cheesecake and put a clean gown on a patient who has just died. I have a callus on the third joint of my middle finger from all those years of writing with a pen before I could afford a computer. Now my hands turn blue when I take ice cubes out of the freezer. Raynaud's Syndrome is the medical term: *severe, paroxysmal, vascular disorder causing disturbances of the circulation in the extremities.*

When I was a student nurse in anatomy class, my hands dissected a cat, felt the difference between striated and smooth muscle, differentiated between femur and ulna. I think of that as I hold Peter in my lap, how this whole cat is so much more beautiful than its parts. As I sit at the computer, these hands help me make sense of my life. My left hand meets my right around my cof-fee cup and together we dream about what they will hold tomorrow. Touch makes the world tolerable.

Life isn't an accumulation of years, but of moments. And moments turn into poems if I let them simmer long enough. All of my writing is about people, how each person is a miracle in mind and memory and intelligence, as well as anatomy and physiology. *Motives. Feelings. Ambitions. Hopes. Disappointments.*

Albert Camus, a twentieth-century, Algerian-born, French philosopher and novelist, wrote in his *Notebooks*, "There is but one freedom…to put oneself right with death. After that everything is possible." (*Notebook V, Sept. 1945-Apr. 1948*, Translated from the French and annotated by Justin O'Brien, New York: Knoppf, 1965, p. 151). Illness is a spiritual flat tire, a reset button, a wake-up call, a disruption that seems like a disaster but can end up redirecting a life in a meaningful way. A new birth. Learning to sing "ability" instead of "disability." Anger, because it gets the person moving, may be a more positive response to a grim diagnosis than passive resignation. Love and healing are possible even when a cure is not. In the twenty years I worked as a registered nurse, I saw miracles happen. The birth of a healthy child after the umbilical cord was wrapped around his neck. An ovarian cyst that magically disappears. A cut-open body somehow magically heals against great odds. The miracle of a fertilized egg grows up into my six-foot-four-inch beautiful son. My body speaks and I've learned to listen, one hour at a time. *Soak in a bubble bath. Trust what feels good. Dress well. Wear makeup every day. Seek the latest medical information about lupus. Pray. Accept support. Let go of the past, of trying to have control of nonessential tasks. Listen to the inner voice of intuition.*

What matters in my life? Sitting on the patio and watching the sun fall behind the Rocky Mountains. My son's laugh. Feeling summer rain on my face. Talking to a friend on the phone. My fireplace. My home, where I've created space for peace and contemplation and a safe place to write. The wind, lake, and ash trees are my community, and I'm part of the landscape. In a world seemingly bent on its own destruction, the act of creation is the only thing that makes sense. *Dare to disturb the universe with your truths. Never settle for less than the impossible.*

The advice often given to writers is, "write about what you know." I believe that an even more important philosophy is to write about what matters. Writing about people caught up in the medical system fills both of these criteria. I write to give voice to patients and family members and doctors and nurses. Writing is an act of faith. *Treat writing as a sacred act. Immerse yourself totally in what you love. Learn to listen to your inner editor.*

Growing up, I read voraciously everything I could get my hands on. *Bobbsey Twins. Nancy Drew. Army Nurse: Cherry Ames.* All the horse and dog stories. My father was a Methodist minister. Hearing the Bible read out loud was the beginning of my love affair with words, the silence between stanzas, the poetry, with the rhythms and music of the *Psalms* and *The Song of Solomon*, the most sensuous love poems ever written.

For me, writing is making sense out of the chaos with which we are constantly bombarded, finding the connection between the unconscious mind and my writing arm, and attempting to make something beautiful out of pain. My work tries to show how it feels to be both nurse and patient, the caregiver and the care receiver, and how difficult it is to be on either side of the medical dilemma.

I write notes in my journal for essays and stories and usually work directly on the computer in these forms. The piece starts to emerge through the revision process, and learning how to rein in the critic in my brain in order for the storyteller to have her say. Learning that these two sides of myself are not at war, but that each has her role in the creative process. Writing is solitude and pushing past weariness to find that hidden reserve of energy, allowing me to finish a poem or essay or story.

Reading is one of life's most mind-expanding pleasures and requires no muscle. I often read books twice: once for the story, and the second time, critically, to examine what works in the book and what doesn't. I read to see what the book can teach me about how to improve my own work, read with critical attention, every faculty alert. My first published poem was written while I was a senior at Illinois College. This poem, about my ill-fated marriage, was written four years before my husband and I separated. Writing has always been the place where I find out what I'm thinking, how I'm feeling. Once it was written, I could no longer deny the true state of my marriage.

I get up, have a cup of coffee, brush my teeth, sit on the chaise lounge in my living room, turn on the laptop and the gas fireplace, and my day has started. I found the antique chaise lounge at a garage sale, a derelict with exposed springs and rain-bleached wood. I refinished the wood and a local artisan restored the upholstery to its former beauty. All I need are my favorite pen and hard-backed journal. Quality staring-out-the-window time. *Drift. Wait. Obey.* Ella Fitzgerald, Miles Davis, Sarah Vaughn on the local jazz station.

Journals help me organize the different projects I'm working on; they hold research notes, my own life story, my rantings about the social injustice I observe in the world, and snippets of dialogue and metaphor that I often end up using when I can find an appropriate spot. Journals help me define themes that I return to in my work: the body and its fallibility, and love in all its forms: parent and child, nurse and patient, man and woman, man and nature.

The creative process is a combination of discipline and hard work and tangential thinking. Often, when I'm cooking dinner or driving the car, I'll suddenly know what I need to do with a piece I was working on that morning. My mind was working on the problem all along. For me, this is the miracle of creativity. I don't believe in writer's block; there's always something that I can revise or research or retype.

Medical journal articles, so full of hard little facts, tell me nothing about the boy lying in intensive care in a diabetic coma, or about the young mother who has suffered a myocardial infarction at twenty-two. I write to give these cold facts a name, a heart, a story, to find the internal hum that turns into stanzas, sentences, paragraphs. I write in hope that my characters will earn birth certificates, get up and walk off the page, happy and healthy, with lives of their own.

POETRY PUBLICATIONS

Studer's poetry publications include the following book:

Prayer to a Purple God. Lewiston, N.Y.: Mellen Poetry, 1996.

Studer has poems published in the following journals:

Balance: The Lifestyle Magazine for Women Physicians; Birmingham Poetry Review; Bloomsbury Review; Calapooya; Caregiving Poetry Review; Collage; Cream City Review; Devil's Millhopper; Disability Rag and Resource; Earth's Daughters; Eclipse; Eleventh Muse; Embers; High Plains Literary Review; International Magazine of Poetry; Kaleidoscope; Mediphors; Midnight Lamp; Minnesota Review; Newsletter Inago; Paris/Atlantic; Sing Heavenly Muse!; The Sun; Zone 3.

Studer's poetry is included in the following anthologies:

Hyperion: Black Sun New Moon. Ed. Judy Hogan. Chapel Hill, N.C.: Carolina Wren Press, 1980.
Prairie Smoke: The Pueblo Poetry Project 1979–1989. Ed. Tony Moffeit. Pueblo, Colo.: Univ. of Southern Colorado Press, 1990.
Toward Solomon's Mountain: The Experience of Disability in Poetry. Ed. Joseph L. Baird and Deborah S. Workman. Philadelphia: Temple Univ. Press, 1986.
We Speak for Peace. Ed. Ruth Harriet Jacobs. Manchester, Conn.: Knowledge, Ideas and Trends (KIT), 1993.
Wingbone: Poetry from Colorado. Ed. Janice Hays and Pamela Haines. Colorado Springs, Colo.: Sudden Jungle, 1987.

Studer has translated Dutch poetry to English in the following anthologies:

The Age of Koestler. Ed. Nicolaus P. Kogon. Kalamazoo, Mich.: Practices of
  the Wind, 1994.
Practices of the Wind. Ed. Nicolaus Waskowsky and David M. Marovich.
  Kalamazoo, Mich.: Practices of the Wind, 1980.

*Studer's Dutch to English poetry translations have been included in the following
journals:*

Blue Buildings; Midnight Lamp; Poetry East; Visions.

Anne Webster

❦

*Going home is an effective and dramatic theme used by many writers, and Web-
ster uses it superbly. The reader will follow her from her childhood on "Bolton
Road" to her domestic life in "The Woman My Husband Should Have Married."
On this metaphoric journey, the reader also learns about her trials with personal
illness and her ability to laugh and enjoy life in spite of the physical symptoms
that sometimes control her body. The names of Doctors Sjögren, Raynaud, and
Crohn have implications beyond the textbook. Webster's sense of humor, com-
bined with her honesty and self-awareness, illustrate that "home" is not so much
a place outside us as a place within.*

THE HOUSE ON BOLTON ROAD

I drive past it on the way to the airport.
Shabby men lounge with their cigarettes
on the front steps. The vast spread of grass
where I once built small towns with acorns
in the roots of an absent fir tree has shrunk
to a weedy strip only yards from the street.
Instead of a rabbit-warren rooming house,
I see the brick fortress, my grandmother
Annie's house, her gift from a mail order groom,
a dirt farmer turned insurance salesman.

I want to turn in the driveway, tell the guys,
"I used to live here. Can I come in and look around?"
I would walk up those steps, past the screen porch
where Annie taught me how to crochet doilies,
through the living room, chairs circled like wagons
around a wood stove, down the long hall,

turn left to the kitchen where a heart attack
took my grandfather, where I sat after school
in first grade listening to Stella Dallas,
watching Annie push her weight into the handle
of a grinder, making meatloaf for supper
while my parents worked downtown.

My big sister and I slept across from the kitchen,
in the room where Annie's parents had died,
the refuge my sister shoved me from when
she heard noises in the night. Again, I tiptoe
down the haunted hall past Annie's snoring,
past Reggie Sue, the boarder, to the front room
to wake our parents. I would find them there,
still beautiful, in their thirties with jet hair,
wrapped in each other's arms, innocent as me
at six of the time when whisky would drive
a stake through the heart of their marriage
and Daddy would sit among men like those
on the steps, trying to warm himself in the sun.

THE DAY OF MY SIXTH birthday and the day after Christmas, I held my new bride doll, fingering the skirt of her white taffeta dress as I stood with my parents by a backyard trash fire. Their voices rumbled over me as they discussed what they would throw away, what they would burn. We were moving, they said, to live with Annie, my father's mother, a few miles away.

My sister Rosemary, five years older, later told me that we had to move because of Daddy's drinking. Did that mean the brown bottles I saw him nipping from, the ones he hid in the trunk of his car, in the hall closet, and between the couch cushions? When I caught him at it, he told me it was his "medicine." I remembered wild rides home from dinners at friends' houses. I had crouched at Mother's feet under the dash while he had careened and swerved, clipping mailboxes as though the drive were some early model for a computer game. Mother and Rosemary had shrieked, my sister clutching Mother's shoulders from the back seat. But the bad driving wasn't the only reason we were moving: Rosemary said that Daddy had "gambled the money away."

Before our move, Mother had cried every night, begging Daddy to quit drinking, and Rosemary had retreated into a sullen place that walled out the voices. I alone had been happy in our first house. The one to most resemble him, I was my father's constant companion. On weekends he took me with him to the business where he sold tires; I played on his adding machine, kicked tires with him, and measured their treads. Other Saturdays we went fishing on the banks of the Chattahoochee, where he patiently baited my hooks and told me stories of our Indian heritage. We dug up our backyard to plant corn in spring and raked leaves together in fall.

After the move, we lived by Annie's stern rules: she didn't tolerate misbehavior by children or adults. Daddy no longer came home drunk or sneaked nips. He and Mother spoke in quiet voices, though Mother sometimes became teary eyed with fatigue from the job she had taken downtown to help pay off his gambling debts. Rosemary and I also knew not to cross Annie; she didn't respond to whining as our parents did.

The big, old brick house my grandfather had built for Annie before the Depression gracefully absorbed our little family. Rosemary and I slept in the back bedroom, the room where my great-grandparents had spent their last years when I was a toddler. My grandfather had died just after my birth, so Annie slept alone in the biggest bedroom. Reggie Sue, a school teacher who boarded with her, lived in the next room down the long hall. Mother and Daddy slept in the front room with the French doors that opened onto the living room. That we all shared one bathroom and one phone—with a party line—never seemed to bother anyone.

During years that we lived there, I was in little-girl heaven. Daddy and I played long games of gin rummy. (He took ten cards to my seven, saying that it gave me a better chance, something I doubted even then.) Annie taught me how to win every game of Chinese checkers, how to tell the future on a Ouija board, and, best of all, how to crochet. She would sit with me, patiently showing me how to form stitches. She was left-handed and I was right-handed, making it impossible for her to put her arms around me and take my hands in hers to demonstrate, but she never flagged until I could produce doilies and dresser scarves.

Solitary playing kept me busy the rest of the time. I learned to roller skate on the cement walk in front of the house. Among the roots of a big fir tree beside the drive, I built cities of acorns and sticks. The chickens pecking in the yard and the woods behind the henhouse provided hours of idle entertainment.

We knew everyone on the street and were kin to many. My great-great-grandfather McDonald had arrived with nine sons in a covered wagon at the end of the Civil War to start a farm a mile away. There were Annie's siblings—Dr. Paul, a general practitioner, and Mark, a retired stained glass cutter, with his wife Mary Lee, plus Annie's double first cousins "Cuddens" Grover, Lily, and Myrtie. (Their parents and Annie's parents had been sisters and identical twin brothers.) I wandered from house to house, equally at home in any of them. The McDonald side of the family doted on me, the smallest child and the one that most resembled them.

Daddy and Annie liked to brag that I looked like a "McDonald," with my straight dark hair and brown eyes. We would hold up our hands, side by side, remarking on how our nails and fingers were similarly shaped, how our olive skins matched, as though we were members of an exclusive club. And indeed we were. That club was the Cherokee Nation. Annie's great grandfather had arrived in Virginia from Scotland in the late eighteenth century to marry a Cherokee woman. Daddy and Annie took more pride in this fact than all of our Scots Irish forebears.

We moved away from Bolton Road to a small house two years later when Daddy's debts were paid. Mother's parents gave them the down payment on a house near them. The house was so small—three rooms—that Rosemary and I slept on a rollaway bed in the kitchen. Mother continued to work, and Daddy not only resumed his drinking, but accelerated it. Within four years my sister would marry at sixteen to escape the alcoholic monster he had become. Mother, with me at eleven her only responsibility, would try to escape through divorce, although divorce would not resolve her depression.

I continued to visit Annie's house, though only in my dreams. Well into my thirties, I often woke after dreaming that I still lived there, the huge house sitting in its broad expanse of lawn as I wandered the rooms that came off the central hallway like limbs of a tree.

The dreams stopped when, at thirty-nine, I moved a couple of miles from Bolton Road. Though the old neighborhood had become a near slum, my route to the airport brought me past the house. The once-handsome home now housed only boarders, rough-looking men who sat on the front steps in mild weather. The large yard with the towering fir and field of jonquils in spring had become hard-packed dirt, only yards wide. Instead of the quiet neighborhood where everyone knew each other, many of the houses had been torn down and heavy trucks rumbled past. Still, that house stood as a symbol of the happiest time of my childhood, and my eyes are drawn to it each time I pass, as if searching for a trace of those golden days.

By writing this poem, I captured some of my past on paper—not only the house, but so many people whom I have loved. With each reading, I have a physical feeling, a twist of my gut, when I picture my parents still young and beautiful, their lives not yet ruined. It helps to ease the memories of my father's quick wit, later dulled by years of alcoholism, of his death by lung cancer after a lifetime of smoking. I can almost experience a moment of peace with my mother's suicide after her decades of depression, brought on in part by her conviction that if she had been a better woman, Daddy would have stopped drinking. In this poem she is "still beautiful."

I believe this poem is a favorite of my readers because it evokes a common theme. We all have childhood memories of a place and people we would like to see once again, memories that we could turn in our hands and examine, free of the constraints of time, as if they were captured in a crystal globe. This poem serves that function for me, and, I hope, my for readers.

Going Steady

Diseases are often named for the doctors
who first catalog their symptoms.

What woman hasn't imagined being
in bed with more than one man?
But a good girl, long married, I was never
into the kinky stuff. Suddenly my fantasy
comes true: three new guys share me.
If it were high school, I would wear
a senior ring caked with wax,
a letterman's jacket, sleeves rolled up,
a fraternity pin over my left tit.
My new lovers, doctors all—
Wouldn't my mother be proud?—
hardly let me get out of bed.
These sexy seducers leave brands
like whisker burns and sucking kisses.

Dr. Sjögren, that charming Swede,
likes to talk nasty: *here's to sand*
in your eyes, my little prune.
Dr. Reynaud, French to the core,
kisses my lilac fingertips, murmuring,
froid hands, chaud heart, ma chère.
Dr. Crohn, a plain-speaking American,
thinks foreplay is whispers of
hot to trot, guts on fire.
These men don't have a jealous bone.
I can still flirt with guys in hard hats

sporting tattoos on rocky biceps.
Lefty Lupus, that old wolf, says
my skin rash turns him on.
His pal, Slammo Sclera D, would like
to lick my smooth knuckles, but for once
I'm too exhausted to think about sex.

After nine years away from nursing, I took a refresher course and ended up working on a cardiac step-down unit, taking care of patients who had undergone angioplasty or bypass surgery. My prior job had been as the nursing administrator for five busy critical-care units, and before that I had worked in both ICU and CCU.

This unit seemed a perfect fit for me. Most of the patients, at fifty-one, were my age or older, and I found an easy camaraderie with the men and their wives, even more so with the occasional woman patient. Any of the people to whom I was assigned could have been one of my friends, and, indeed, I sometimes reported to work to find someone I knew—once a man from my writing group, another time, a second cousin.

This kind of nursing had yet another benefit I hadn't expected. Unlike my friends and family, these people, laid low by heart disease, eagerly listened to my lectures on diet and exercise.

My obsession with food had begun twenty years earlier when I had read Adele Davis's *Let's Get Well.* Using her book as my bible, I had served my protesting family raw sugar, whole grain breads, and liver until everyone groaned when I brought up the subject of healthy eating. As if to prove me wrong, my husband Larry often existed for days on only shiny white and brown food—refined starches and meat coated with fat. He thought himself excused from diet worries by his thirty-two inch waistline. I quizzed him daily. "How many servings of vegetables have you had today? Any fruit?" He would only grunt in answer.

I counted my daily portions—five veggies, three fruits, two dairy, and two proteins, plus several of whole grains. Only after I'd eaten my quota of the healthy stuff would I allow myself a cookie or a glass of wine. My reputation for being "a food nut" led to my friends warily calling to ask about the menu when I invited them to dinner, as if they were afraid of low-fat poisoning.

"Just being around you makes me want to eat something bad," my daughter-in-law once told me. In the break room the other nurses pretended to admire my lunch choices. "Oh, look. Anne is eating something *healthy,*" one might say, peering at my plate of four vegetables. In contrast, my colleagues would dig into hamburgers, French fries, and saucer-sized cookies. And they, of all people, knew better.

Proper diet wasn't the only thing I preached. "I've had the best week ever," I once told Larry. "I ran twenty-five miles, lifted weights four hours, and did three step classes." I believed that, along with good food, exercise could conquer any physical problem, except, perhaps, cancer.

I took no chances. Along with my diet and exercise regimen, I took a fistful of supplements. Fortified with all the vitamins of the alphabet and small boulders of heavy minerals like calcium, magnesium, and zinc, my body was as protected as a hillside fortress.

I hated to admit that my mother motivated my good intentions, and that my obsession with healthy living had begun with her suicide. The first time I had realized her pervasive influence had been when, at thirty-seven, I began seeing a therapist. Though it had been two years since my parents had died, I couldn't shed my grief. I had found myself studying the obituaries, imagining my own name in the bold print and how people would read of my untimely death and sigh. My usual enthusiasm and pleasure in small things disappeared, leaving me almost sleepwalking through my days.

Daddy had died four months after Mother, with pneumonia bubbling in his diseased lungs. He and I had not been close for many years, so his death hadn't been as difficult as Mother's for me to accept. However, the loss of both of them had pulled me down until I felt as though I were drowning

During therapy I learned to let go of that grief. I also came to realize that my unconscious resolve not to repeat Mother's physical decline was what drove me in my search for health. Overweight and out of shape, she had limped around with a cane at the end, constantly complaining of pain. Her poor physical condition, coupled with lifelong depression, had contributed to her decision to die.

Though I understood my motivation intellectually, that knowledge had done nothing to influence my obsession with health and my determinedly cheerful demeanor—depression was a word too frightening to consider. Those traits remained as much as part of me as the stripes on a tabby cat. As long as I could do everything I or others asked of me, I was safe from a fate like Mother's.

About the same time I went back to work, I began to have physical symptoms.

My fingers often turned an unflattering shade of lavender. When I first noticed the discoloration, I thought I had used a leaky pen, but soon I realized it was a circulatory problem, probably Raynaud's, that left my hands icy and blue. It only bothered me when I had to touch patients. "Lord, honey, I pity your husband!" one patient said when I reached under the covers to check his pedal pulses.

Soon I woke each morning with hands that had become claws. No matter how I tried, I couldn't make a fist until I'd been up twenty minutes or so and had warmed them around a mug of coffee. The stiffness was joined by pains in the small joints of my fingers and toes, pains that migrated as I tried to sleep at night until I was tempted to peek under the covers to see if they were sending out sparks. Add chronic knee pain (too much running and squatting heavy weight), tennis elbow (tendonitis from too much tennis), and cervical-nerve root impingement (years of carrying a heavy shoulder bag), and I was an arthritic mess. But I took ibuprofen, ignoring those pains it didn't relieve. At work I was too busy to notice the discomfort.

Finally my doctor sent me to a rheumatologist. I went gladly, sure that he could prescribe something to stop the nuisance. After all, proactive was my middle name. He told me that I had features of scleroderma, accompanied by lupus and Sjögren's syndrome. In as deep denial as mine, my internist told me not to worry, that I was healthy, and to forget my next appointment with the specialist.

Four years after that nursing refresher course, I loved going to work. At fifty-five, I was the oldest nurse in my unit, but I took pride in my youthful vigor. Sure, I got tired at work, but many twenty-five-year-old nurses dragged around worse than I did.

"What are you smiling about?" my colleagues often asked me.

"Oh, I'm just happy to be here," I would answer. I fed on the adrenalin of taking care of high-risk people. So what if my hands turned blue in the air conditioning when I was charting? I just twisted around on my stool and kept them out of sight. If I had a little arthritis in my neck and knees, I wasn't going to advertise it—certainly not to these babies.

When work left me too tired to cook, I didn't complain. It would be the same as admitting that I was too old for my job. Besides, if I whined at home, I knew exactly what Larry would say: "Quit that damn job if it bothers you. We don't need the money." So I made myself act perky in the evenings and put dinner on the table with a smile, even if weariness hung over my shoulders like a lead stole.

On my off days, I sent poems out to literary magazines, completed business writing lessons for students in the correspondence course that I taught, and went to the gym for my daily aerobic fix. On the weekends I played with my little grandsons and had dinner with friends. My life couldn't have been better, and to keep it that way, I took perfect care of myself, or so I thought. I kept running on my hamster wheel, thinking I would somehow keep ahead of the clock.

Still, my arthritis symptoms steadily worsened, and I began to have frequent GI upsets. Never mind that I saw fresh blood in my stools on occasion—I had self-diagnosed this as internal hemorrhoids. Weren't hemorrhoids almost an occupational hazard for nurses? Never mind that my red blood count had been low for the past year. Perhaps I needed to adjust my protein intake.

Finally my internist sent me for a second opinion. The new rheumatologist disagreed with what the first had said, saying that I didn't have lupus. I felt relieved, vindicated, until she said, "Not only do you have Raynaud's and Sjögren's, I believe you have inflammatory bowel disease accompanied by a systemic arthritis."

A colonoscopy soon confirmed her diagnosis. Crohn's disease was something I had rarely seen, and then it had been in thin, pasty people who often ran for the bathroom—not vigorous, healthy people like me. Though I told Larry that I would give it six weeks until I would be okay, the symptoms returned more viciously than before. I had to call off from work so often that, after six months of frequent absences, my charge nurse told me to stay home. My doctors concurred: no more nursing for me.

Soon I was able to be out of bed for only hours at a time, taking larger and larger doses of steroids. I lay on top of the covers, my head buzzing, as I missed my colleagues and patients, my trips to the gym, and my old, active life. No longer could I romp with my two toddler grandsons or take the long walks I craved.

Over the next year, I gradually resumed many activities, but at a pace that my body dictated. If I tried to skip my hour rest after lunch, my symptoms increased; total exhaustion, multiple joint pains, and a belly ache would set in as if they had been waiting for an offstage cue. As I began to understand that I would never go back to work, that I would never be able to lead the busy life I had loved, I became angry and, yes, depressed. It took me another two years to go through the grieving process, to learn to appreciate each day that I felt well, and to be happy with a slower-paced existence.

"Going Steady" is a favorite poem of mine because it embodies the new me, the person who can laugh at her illness. Those physical symptoms that once dismayed me—even to the occasional exhaustion of the last line—may sometimes control my body, but never my joy in living.

TRUE COLORS

My husband phones me from Costa Rica
in the shadow of the Arenal Volcano,
a growling monster I can hear thousands
of miles distant over crackling wire.
He describes chunks of molten rock
big as box cars bouncing down the hillside,
a night sky lit by flames, bubbling lava rivers
and—click—he is gone, the phone dead.

At work I am thinking of him when Mr. Dolan,
a coronary bypass patient I had just seen,
turns on the call light. I find a canyon
in his chest, an infected sternal wound
laid open by festered muscle, rotted sutures.
A wayward finger of bypassed artery
waves free; the walls sparkle, sprayed
gang-war red. Mr. Dolan's dead eyes stare.

My husband comes home to me unsinged,
but I am scarred, as if by Arenal.
I tiptoe around boiling pots, honed blades,
drive slowly in the right-hand lane.
Mr. Dolan visits my dreams to remind me
of my own pulsing lava, the hidden rainbow
palate—goldenrod fat, damson spleen,
lilac intestine—and the price of opening
this thin skin sack to my own scalding beauty.

When one hears the term "true colors," one probably thinks about a person showing what they're made of or their true worth—like someone who is "spineless" or someone who has "a stiff upper lip." When I literally saw inside someone during surgery, the meaning of that term changed forever.

I was eighteen, in my second year of nursing school, when I began my surgery rotation. I had already learned to bathe, catheterize, and give injections, but the prospect of working in the OR as a scrub nurse, passing instruments and seeing people's insides, made me feel like an infantry recruit going into battle. I was eager to be initiated into that secret society, but would I disgrace myself?

The first operation that I scrubbed on was in inguinal herniorrhaphy. I had held my breath as the surgeon slid the scalpel in a diagonal path across the patient's groin. Blood rose in a thick line, but I was soon too busy handing the doctor clamps and sponges to think about getting sick, even when the Bovie cautery sent up puffs of smoke smelling of cooked flesh.

Abdominal surgeries became Technicolor magic. A doctor would plunge his hands into a belly, pull out ropey intestines, and lay them on sterile towels beside the incision. After suctioning away excess blood, he would point out a stomach, liver, or spleen in the dark well of an abdominal cavity. Against the deep red muscle, the softer colors of the organs seemed to glow—shiny lilac, wet maroon, subtle pinks, and the brassy yellow of fat. I often sighed with happiness. How many people got to see inside a living body, to help with an operation?

After my three-month assignment in the operating room, it would be almost twenty years before I saw a person's organs again, but this time the patient would be awake. I had been on duty on the evening shift in the emergency room of a downtown hospital. Because our hospital was near the big trauma center, we rarely saw patients with major injuries. I was working a crossword puzzle when an ambulance driver shoved the glass doors open, carrying a large carton marked "O Positive blood." He told me that he had a patient from a distant small town and that the man had gas gangrene. What was he talking about? A wound treated as an emergency would never be old enough to have become gangrenous. If it hadn't been for the box of blood, I would have snickered. When another driver arrived pushing a stretcher with blood streaming off of the sides, I came to attention.

The patient, a big-boned African American man, returned my greeting. When I asked if I could examine him, the patient clutched at the sheet over his chest, as if embarrassed. I could hardly believe his injury: loops of intestines spilled out of his lower abdomen onto the stretcher. Unlike the clean and shiny intestines I had seen in surgery so long ago, large clots studded them. "Are you in pain?" I asked.

"Just a little," he said, pointing to a nick in an upper eyelid. "I was changing a truck tire, and the jack slipped. The wheel rim caught me."

The man lay quietly as I gloved up and covered the exposed organs in sterile saline and gauze. I kept reassuring him that he would be okay, as much for my sake as his. We made small talk until he went to surgery. He didn't have to say that he did hard physical labor—his heavily muscled arms and callused hands attested to a lifetime of it, as did his uncomplaining stoicism while he waited for the OR crew.

For weeks the image of his butchered abdomen spilling those intestines, of his inky, trusting eyes, haunted me. I later learned that he had survived the surgery without an infection, but that the trauma had led to kidney failure, which had killed him.

Twenty years later I took care of another patient who would remind me again of the danger of exposing the beauty that lies inside each of us. Mr. Dolan had been my patient in the cardiac step-down unit after his coronary bypass surgery. I came to work after a couple of days off to find that he had not gone home as expected, but had developed a sternal-wound infection. My husband had gone to Costa Rica with a buddy, and I had been looking forward to a rare weekend on the evening shift rather than the frantic routine of the day shift, that is, until I heard about Mr. Dolan.

I had taken care of a few infected sternal wounds, and I dreaded it. I knew too well the hot, rotting smell of dead flesh. But worse would be the painful treatment. I would have to pack it with gauze impregnated with an antibiotic.

When the drug touched the raw incision, it burned like acid, as one patient had described it. Although I had long ago become inured to the sight of almost any incision, inflicting pain on a patient could make me woozy.

"Bear with me while I redress your wound," I told Mr. Dolan. I had to stop myself from flinching when I saw the huge hole in his chest. As in the other such infections I had seen, the incision had begun to split and part, but never as widely as this one. Six or eight inches long, the puffy edges stood at least four inches apart.

I used forceps to pull out ropes of pus-streaked gauze, trying not to let my expression reflect how the dead-animal odor turned my stomach. The angry walls of the incision stood another three inches deep, and at the bottom, just over the pericardial sac, pooled globs of creamy yellow pus that bounced with each heartbeat. "I have to pack the wound with an antibiotic, and it will hurt for a few minutes," I said. Despite my warning, Mr. Dolan barked in pain when the antibiotic touched him. We both gritted our teeth until I finally finished.

At the desk, intent on blocking out the image of Mr. Dolan's chest, I thought about my husband Larry and his phone call of the night before. Larry had been describing the Arenal Volcano, telling me how flames shot up a hundred feet in the air and boulders the size of school buses rolled down the mountain side. "It sounds like a shotgun. Can you hear it?" was the last thing he said before the line went dead. Although I had joked to the other nurses that my husband might be fried to a crisp, I felt an edge of nervousness.

As I checked on my patients just before going home, Mr. Dolan lay sleeping; the light from the hall showed his face finally relaxed. After I had done his initial dressing, a plastic surgeon had come to evaluate him for wound closure. That doctor had yanked out my gauze, so that I had to pack the wound yet another time. Mr. Dolan deserved some rest.

The next afternoon when I reported for duty, the day nurse greeted me with the bad news: "Mr. Dolan died last night." She told me that the night nurse had found him unconscious at 12:30 A.M. She described blood covering the bed, the floor, and the walls. "One of his grafted coronary arteries must have rotted through, and he pumped like a geyser until he was empty."

Larry came home unscorched a few days later, but my faith in living had been cracked, as if by an aftershock of Mr. Dolan's death. I kept imagining his blood all over the room, reminded anew of how exposure of parts not meant to be seen could end a person's life. I thought again of my OR experience, how the muted rose and lilac of the intestines had rested in shining white fascia and golden fat. Their beauty was, like the hot reds and oranges of a volcano's boiling lava, often deadly when exposed to the human eye. Those vivid images led me to write the poem as if I had actually been the one to find Mr. Dolan in his blood-splattered room.

Losing a patient like Mr. Dolan reminded me yet again that death can come suddenly and unexpectedly and that writing could help me survive being a witness to it.

I have learned that writing is a way for me to cope with difficult emotions, to keep them from sucking me under to depression. I began to trust that through writing, painful events could become life experiences to be shared with others. By the time of Mr. Dolan's death, I had come to rely on turning the pain of such situations into a written record, something outside of myself.

THE WOMAN MY HUSBAND SHOULD HAVE MARRIED

I know exactly what she looks like: big, perky
breasts, tight, little waist and long blonde hair.
This woman likes to cook. Every night she
serves him a feast of fresh vegetables, fried
chicken or steak, minus the lectures about arteries
slamming shut. Her idea of fun is watching him
ride his tractor around their farm in south
Georgia where she sews and makes preserves
when not entertaining his relatives. She knows
all the rules of baseball and football, likes to
watch golf on TV with him Sunday afternoons.

He cannot hurt her feelings. His sexist jokes
make her laugh until tears run. She squeezes
a dollar until it stretches like rubber, never
runs up the credit cards, not her. She dresses
like a queen in last year's clothes, always
wearing the three-inch heels he loves. She won't
let him help in the kitchen and rubs his back
when the dishes are done. She hates foreplay:
she lies back, wet and ready in ten seconds flat,
unless, of course, he prefers a blow job.

Poor guy. He got me instead. A city girl,
who lives for books, art, long slow kisses,
who hates cooking and sports. Once,

when I was gone a month, friends gave him
a blow-up doll. Now, when he walks in
that door, his pink face full of hope, I want
to be that doll, Marilyn Monroe in an apron,
waiting for the details of his golf game.
Instead I quietly leave him with his TV
and newspaper so he can at least pretend.

Larry and I married on a Saturday afternoon in September, four days after I finished nursing school. We had timed our wedding so that I could return to Auburn University with him when he began his coursework the next week for his final quarter. I was twenty and he would turn twenty-two in a couple of weeks.

As far as we knew, we had everything in common. Our families both had their roots in rural farming. Larry's parents had grown up scratching a living from the land, as my grandparents had. Our world consisted of rigid Bible Belt rules that propelled us toward youthful marriage—the alternative would have been to burn in hell. We both wanted a better life than that of our parents, and our educations provided us a way. Our vision of the future was that of a couple with 2.5 children, happily living the good life as seen in magazines and on TV.

I had purposely chosen a man different from my father: Larry's steady calm and his rocklike dependability shone like gold against Daddy's mercurial swings between effervescent charm and brutal drunkenness. Where Daddy, darkly handsome, was as reliable as the weather, Larry, blonde and blue eyed, would keep his promise to always be there for me. He had an education—two college degrees, the first in his family ever to graduate college—and the ambition to carry him forward. I never stopped to think why Larry had picked me of all the girls he knew—I just knew I had done the right thing in marrying him.

When we moved into the married students' apartments at Auburn, he had already signed up for flight school in the Marine Corps. I had no further plans in life than beautifying our little apartment and learning to cook the cream pies and chicken and dumplings that he loved. The future meant following my pilot husband from base to base and getting a job at a local hospital if he were assigned anywhere long enough for me to work.

Beyond that I couldn't imagine anything. The women's magazines touted the importance of a strong woman behind every successful man. I had vague images of setting a lovely table for dinner parties for Larry and his business colleagues, of walking through a house—one in which I had chosen every item to reflect our good taste. The thought of children never formed, except as something I wanted to delay thinking about for at least five years.

Two months after our wedding, I found myself pregnant. Larry didn't like condoms, and I thought I had the rhythm method down cold. I had been wrong. After his graduation from Auburn in December, I fought nausea as we moved to Pensacola for his flight training. Any idea I might have had about working had to wait on the baby.

Our son John was born in Mississippi while Larry was stationed at the jet base in Meridian. Several moves later brought us to South Carolina, where he received orders to join a marine squadron flying off of a navy carrier. I moved to Alabama to live with his parents while he was gone so that they could care for John while I worked at a local hospital.

The first hint I had of our differences came when Larry was flying touch-and-go landings off of the USS Forrestal in the Mediterranean. In his letters he admitted to fear—one of the few times he would do so—at night landings. He spoke of the black seas and trying to put his plane down in the dark on something "like a moving postage stamp."

In his absence I had spent the lonely evenings with books that I thought would help to complete my one-sided nursing-school education. I read up on art and philosophy, especially on twentieth-century French philosopher Sartre's existentialism and English philosopher Russell's atheism. When I wrote to him of my excitement at realizing that there were other worldviews outside our narrow upbringing, he shot back a letter, saying to "forget that crap and get down on your knees to pray for me." It was the beginning of a long battle over his disdain for what he called "big-headed intellectuals."

Those differences grew over the years. Larry craved physical action—golf, tennis, and skiing. His choice of reading consisted of magazines and periodicals, with the occasional thriller thrown into the mix. In the movies he liked, "something happened," usually something violent or involving a car chase. I went with him to tennis matches when I would rather have been browsing galleries, going to plays, or seeing the latest European film with subtitles. Once, when reading a volume of Anne Sexton's poems, I told Larry that I felt as if I were electrically charged. "I've never felt anything like that," he responded.

He also resented the fact that I insisted on working since his job as an airline pilot provided a generous salary. Larry would come home from a four-day trip, only to have me wave at him on my way to the hospital to do an evening shift. The weekends that I often had to work seemed to fall on the ones he had off. Yet I couldn't give up either my job or my ambition.

We learned accommodations over the years. I went to meetings of my writing groups, on trips to New York to see art and theater, and to Germany for language courses. He went skiing with old marine buddies and on golf trips to the British Isles.

At the core of our relationship were our shared values—raising our children, building a home, always placing our life together ahead of other distractions. We finally came to rely on each other for our different bodies of knowledge. If I wanted to know about a world leader or where some small island lay, I asked him. He would ask me about artists and literary references from his reading.

I always felt a little sorry for him. Such a wonderful man, and what did he get? Not the ever-smiling wife who loved to cook, who would move to the sticks where he could have some land and maybe a tractor, who never argued about feminist issues. I knew that somewhere he harbored a fantasy of coming home to an immaculate house filled with the aroma of good cooking, to a wife who agreed happily with his political pronouncements, to a sexual partner who didn't demand equal time. He got me instead—an edgy and often uncompromising person who was always looking for that something more intellectual, who was hooked on city living.

The poem is a favorite of mine because, in this little way, I give him the woman of his dreams. And I compose her in my own words.

POETRY PUBLICATIONS

Webster has poems published in the following journals:

Cedar Hills Review; DeKalb Literary Arts Journal; Dream International Quarterly; Explicit Lyrics; Full Moon; Gladstone; I Have Marks to Make; Mediphors; Nebo; New York Quarterly; Solana; Southern Poetry Review; Stony Lonesome; Sunstone Review; 13th Moon; White Crow.

Webster's poetry is included in the following anthologies:

The Ethnic American Woman: Problems, Protests, Lifestyle. Ed. Edith Blicksilver. Debuque, Iowa: Kendall/Hunt, 1978.
Intensive Care: More Poetry and Prose by Nurses. Ed. Cortney Davis and Judy Schaefer. Iowa City: Univ. of Iowa Press, 2003.
O! Georgia: A Collection of Georgia's Newest and Most Promising Writers. Ed. Terri Pepper Galvulic. Cumming, Ga.: Humpus Bumpus, 1999.
Stories of Illness and Healing: Women Write their Bodies. Ed. Sayantani Dasgrupta and Marsha Hurst. Kent, Ohio: Kent State Univ. Press, 2005.

Permissions and Acknowledgments

⁊ઝ

JEANNE BRYNER

"Coal Miner, Caples, WV, 1938" from *Getting By: Stories of Working Lives.*
"In Praise of Hands" from *Tenderly Lift Me* (Kent, Ohio: Kent State Univ. Press, 2004).
"Siderails" from *Journal of Holistic Nursing.*

CORTNEY DAVIS

"Everything in Life Is Divided" from *Bellevue Literary Review* 4:1 (Spring 2004). By permission of Cortney Davis.
"Everything in Life Is Divided" from *Leopold's Maneuvers* (Lincoln: Univ. of Nebraska, 2004).
"The Good Nurse" from *Details of Flesh* (Corvallis, Ore.: Calyx, 1997).
"Heroics" from *American Journal of Nursing.* By permission of *American Journal of Nursing.*
"How I'm Able to Love" from *Leopold's Maneuvers* (Lincoln: Univ. of Nebraska Press, 2004).
"How I'm Able to Love" from *Poetry Magazine.*
"The Nurse's Pockets" from *Between the Heartbeats* (Iowa City: Univ. of Iowa Press, 1995).

THEODORE DEPPE

"Admission, Children's Unit," "The Funeral March of Adolf Wölfi," and "The Japanese Deer," from *The Wanderer King* (Farmington, Maine: Alice James Books, 1996).
"For Don Corleone in Paradise" and "Marisol" from *Cape Clear: New and Selected Poems* (Ireland: Salmon Books, 2002).

SANDRA BISHOP EBNER

"My Father's Violin," "Size 8 Surgical Gloves," "The Cure," and "Motion and Time and Driving Alone" from *The Space Between* (Newtown, Conn.: Hanover Press, 2000).

"Autopsy No. 24722" from *Intensive Care* (Iowa City: Univ. of Iowa Press, 2003).

AMY HADDAD

"Asking for Direction" from *The Arduous Touch* (West Lafayette, Ind.: Purdue Univ. Press, 1999).

"Chemotherapy Lounge" from the *Journal of General Internal Medicine* 19:6 (June 2004).

"Dehiscence" from *Between the Heartbeats* (Iowa City: Univ. of Iowa Press, 1995).

"Girding for Battle" from *Fetishes.*

VENETA MASSON

"La Muerte" from the *Journal of Medical Humanities.*

"Metastasis" and "The Silence of Dollhood" from the *International Journal of Human Caring.*

"The Secret Life of Nurses" from *Nursing and Health Care Perspectives.*

LIANNE MERCER

"Benedición" from *The Healing Environment Without and Within* (G.B.: Royal College of Physicians, 2003).

"Exiles" from *American Journal of Nursing.*

MARY JANE NEALON

"Human-Headed Bull below Empty Space," "The Priesthood," "Rapture," and "Who Dies of Thirst" from *Immaculate Fuel* (New York: Four Way Books, 2004).

Geri Rosenzweig

"Calypso's Bar" from *Pearl.*
"Crossing the Field" from *Nebraska Review.*
"Flaxen God" from *Antigonish Review.*
"This Bach Cantata" from *The Cape Rock.*

Judy Schaefer

"Mathematics" from *Academic Medicine.* By permission of *Academic Medicine.*
"Who Owns the Libretto?" from *Between the Heartbeats* (Iowa City: Univ. of Iowa Press, 1995).

Paula Sergi

"Four on a Fold" from *Boomer Girls* (Iowa City: Univ. of Iowa Press, 1999).
"Germination" from *Rattlewind.*
"Home Visits" and "On Switching from Nursing to English" from *Intensive Care* (Iowa City: Univ. of Iowa Press, 2003).
"Lake de Neveu" from *The Sow's Ear Poetry Review.*

Another version of Sergi's commentary has appeared in the *American Journal of Nursing* by permission of the *American Journal of Nursing.*

Kelly Sievers

"Biopsy" from *Permanente Journal.*
"Holding On" from *Calapooya Collage 16.*
"I Dream Gene Kelly Is My Father" from *Prairie Schooner.*
"In the House across the Street a Boy Is Playing a Horn" from *Seattle Review.*
"Outside the Hotel DeVille" from *Poet Lore,* Special Issue on Visual Art.
"Rochester, Minnesota, 1965" from *The Bridge.*
"Rochester, Minnesota, 1965" from *Between the Heartbeats* (Iowa City: Univ. of Iowa Press, 1995).

KATHLEEN WALSH SPENCER

"Army Nurses, Vietnam, 1966" from *Intensive Care* (Iowa City: Univ. of
    Iowa Press, 2003).
"At the $3 Car Wash" from *Terminus*.
"Coffee for One" from *Lungfull*.
"Sailor Explains Kissing the Nurse" from *MacGuffin*.

CONSTANCE STUDER

"Dear Dr. Williams, Dear Poet" from *Zone 3*.

ANNE WEBSTER

"True Colors" from *Mediphors*.